T0336328

HEALING RHYTHMS
TO
RESET WELLNESS

DR. FRANK LAWLIS

A SAVIO REPUBLIC BOOK
An Imprint of Post Hill Press
ISBN: 978-1-64293-489-2
ISBN (eBook): 978-1-64293-490-8

Healing Rhythms to Reset Wellness
© 2020 by Dr. Frank Lawlis
All Rights Reserved

Cover Design by Cody Corcoran

SAVIO
REPVBLIC
posthillpress.com
New York • Nashville
Published in the United States of America

To my wife, Susan, my life partner and
source of passion and creativity.

CONTENTS

FOREWORD

by Dr. Phil McGraw

When Dr. Frank Lawlis told me about *Healing Rhythms to Reset Wellness*, I asked him if I might have the privilege of writing the foreword to this important work that I know will live on, impacting society for generations to come. He offers works of magnitude, not frivolity, not pop psychology, not trends. He writes about things that strike at the core of our humanness—and this book is no exception.

We have been working together for fifty-plus years: First, at University of North Texas when Dr. Lawlis was my mentor and PhD director in clinical and behavioral medicine programs; later, as colleagues at the groundbreaking trial-science firm Courtroom Sciences; and ultimately, on the *Dr. Phil* show for eighteen years and counting, where he has served in many capacities including chairman of the advisory committee. In everything he does, Dr. Lawlis's impact has been profound.

During all this time, he has always been doing research, finding innovative ways of creating patterns of health for many diseases and mental disorders. At last count, he has written eighteen books and more than a hundred articles on methodologies and studies, which have received awards, and many have become classics. As an innovator, Dr. Lawlis's discoveries and inventions are at least ten years ahead of his time.

When I reviewed *Healing Rhythms to Reset Wellness*, I was struck with his vision for what could be the next era in health for our nation's benefit, which would far surpass the problematic system we have today. This book reaches into ancient wisdoms of healing, to the beginnings of recorded history, and extends these principles into the far futures of tomorrow. It embraces the underlying powers of knowledge we have about what the history of physical, psychological, and spiritual realms of healing mean for the human spirit.

He references the successes of using rhythms by cultures long ago, discusses string theory in quantum physics, and shares space-age knowledge of energy that keeps our galaxy balanced because these elements are related to patterns within the human body and mind. From Plato and Aristotle to Einstein, Dr. Lawlis shows his depth of understanding to translate for us the alignment of powerful forces of nature for wellness through the spheres of consciousness.

This deeply considered articulation of a thesis for healing touches our lives in every aspect. It honors the struggles of our ancestors for the survival of humanity, our inheritance of this DNA strength, and our instinctual need to grow stronger to pass more to our children, grandchildren, and humanity. I believe that Dr. Frank Lawlis expresses a genius in this book that will play a role in each and every life on this planet.

INTRODUCTION

The definition of health should not be the absence of disease,
but the actualization of our potential.

Looking back at my life path, I can see that all the twists and turns it took were determined by discoveries about healing. My passion for them seems to have begun at birth, as a doctor brought me back to life after I was declared dead from complications. He also diagnosed me with severe brain damage that would likely kill me before long. All I knew, growing up, was that this worked in my favor because each stage of my development was celebrated with great fanfare, such as tying my shoes and eating with the right tools.

The lesson from my childhood was that, while I did have neurological challenges, I was able to deal with and overcome those deficits because I was raised by loving family who shared their time, effort, and patience as we worked with my learning problems. One of my early issues with arithmetic was that I simply could not see columns of numbers. So Mom would have me write each problem on a single sheet of paper. My sister taught me to share ideas through writing by acting as reporters and typing out short stories for the newspaper about the adventures of the mysterious Frank Lawlis. One of my heroes was my uncle, who was a physician. He shared his medical books with me and would teach me about the dynamics of medicine. The progress I made as a child with challenges did not come from traditional medical treatments; it was due to the caring determination of the people around me.

My mother suffered more challenging health than I did. Our lives were centered around her illnesses and surgeries. I counted twenty-six surgeries and special programs that were paced so she could maintain a teaching job she loved and, over the years, she greatly influenced many students. My father explained that each new treatment she underwent was necessary, due to past illnesses. Helping care for her and bring her back to daily functioning, over and over again, captured my attention and curiosity. As friends and extended family combined our efforts to bring her back to health, yet again, the question that always remained with me was: *Why couldn't the science of medicine help my mother?*

When I contracted measles at nine years old, pretty much on purpose so I could stay at home, I had an extremely high fever and could not walk steadily. I overheard some dreadful words as the doctor spoke with my parents. He said he would order an iron lung the next day if there was no change. I prayed all night long and asked God how I could heal myself. A message came through that I should "allow" my body to cure itself and I felt assured that I would be all right. The next day, I was dressed to go to school before my parents awoke. I never missed a day of school after that.

These influences led me to eventually receive a PhD in a specialty of psychology I refer to as "medical psychology." I taught in five different medical schools and focused on physical rehabilitation, psychiatry, oncology, and orthopedic surgery to study the healing abilities of the patients I served. I didn't want to compete with existing medical care; my hope was to better integrate the healing experience by researching what happens when we allow the body-mind system to balance itself with love, care, and innate wisdom.

As I enthusiastically entered the field of medical instruction, bitter facts became apparent, which I'll share in Chapter 1. It was my naïve belief that medical schools were supposed to teach the most effective healing approaches, but it dawned on me that the real purpose is to educate future physicians in the traditional practices of the profession. This standard leaves out a lot of wisdom about healing and limits the contributions of other professionals in the business of alleviating suffering, such as psychologists like me. This narrow role would have sufficed if I had seen the limited view behind this American system working successfully. Instead, I made use of clinical experience to observe our innate healing abilities up close.

I learned a lot from watching parents, who are the most instinctual of all healers, with ill children. I watched children who were going through the horrific, but necessary, treatment of severe burn injuries be profoundly calmed by listening to the rhythms of their mother's heartbeat and feeling rocking motions as they were put to sleep. I watched the healing effects of parents stroking their children while they endured the demands of chemotherapy in a war with their cancer. When parents modeled a rhythmic breathing pattern I taught them, children were able to undergo the repeated spinal taps required for their treatment. And when we played specific sound rhythms, autistic children and adults could manage heightened anxiety as they expanded their known, and safe, boundaries in our clinic to engage a bigger world.

As a consultant to an insurance firm in Japan, I found that dancing rhythmically was the most effective way to reduce a serious disease the Japanese call *karoshi*, which means "death from work stress." While I worked to establish stress-management skills with the latest technology, the most successful was a dance exercise. I taught the shuffle step, shifting from one foot to the next, and rocking back and forth to the beat of Brent Lewis's drumming on the album *Primitive Truth*. It was so effective that they scheduled a convention each year and invited five hundred to one thousand people to gather together and dance most of the time. It was exciting to me, because I could see large-scale results from an ancient healing practice.

My quest to study rhythm as a basis for healing came out of a surprising result. I was co-directing a pain clinic for people whose spinal pain was continuing despite traditional medical drugs, surgeries, and therapies. All the skills I had learned in psychotherapy were failing to help them. I had been convinced that hypnosis techniques, highly tuned therapeutic wisdom, and strong diagnostic abilities would cure their pain. I grew so discouraged that I decided to resign, but like other instances in my life, what I needed was a change in my thinking and the intellectual system I was using to approach the problem.

This change occurred when I attended a shamanic workshop with Michael Harner. A shaman is a spiritual leader of a tribe who has special skills and knowledge for healing their health problems. I was fascinated by the material, so after class I asked Michael how he healed spinal pain.

He smiled sheepishly and said, "Frank, you need to learn to play the drum."

And I did. The next week, I asked the patients to sit in a circle. With a brief instruction to relax and listen, I picked up my drum and began beating it in the rhythm I had learned. I continued for only twenty minutes. After, there was an immediate response from an astonished group of patients. They rated their pain as resolved or significantly improved. We continued this regularly and their hope for a return to health was ignited. I felt rhythms could very well be a source of balance for our whole being.

MY RESEARCH AND DISCOVERY

As a natural scientist, and with young psychologists looking for dissertation ideas, I asked a student to collect brain map data from EEGs to study the effects of drumming. We would play different rhythms from cultures around the world—such as Hawaiian, Native American, Japanese, and African—to people with various illnesses and measure the impacts the drumming had on their bodies and emotional states. For example, we played rhythms to cancer patients, looked at the effects on their immune factors, and discovered the ones that made a big difference. The results were clear: Drumming created a marked decrease in anxiety and an upsurge of deep relaxation (theta) states. Later, we discovered an increase in endorphins, which are our body's natural painkillers, when we drummed as surgery was conducted. Since then, my studies have continued in ever more nuanced and targeted ways.

This deep dive into the power of sound to affect brainwaves led me to invent a device called the Bio-Acoustical Utilization

Device (BAUD). It has been approved by the FDA as a biofeedback device that a person can use to discover what frequencies have beneficial effects. For example, in depression, brain maps show that there is an asymmetry of stimulation between the two sides of the brain. The auditory frequencies emitted by BAUD stimulate the brain in certain ways to level both sides up. I'll describe this device more fully in Chapter 3.

With these discoveries and advances, the potential of rhythms to ease the suffering of human beings and increase their thriving struck me so profoundly that I wove a web of explorations into specific practices, applications, and technologies throughout the complexity of our experiences. My passion lies in an ever-deepening understanding of the role of rhythms in life, and I am dedicated to harnessing them as essential components of healing.

WHAT YOU WILL LEARN IN THIS BOOK

This book promises to share ways of healing through rhythms. My hope is that many of them can be integrated within your life and within medical professions as ways of stimulating a whole-being rebalancing effect in cells, tissues, and even emotions that are no longer dancing in step with the rest of the body-mind system. These rhythms can enhance the delivery of medicines to our organs in ways that increase their efficacy.

There are three parts to *Healing Rhythms to Reset Wellness.* Part I shares the philosophical basis for this approach, wisdom that has been around throughout recorded history, as it integrates a view that expands healing beyond illness management. Part II addresses specific health imbalances you may have, which we all face in the course of our lives: sleeplessness, pain, sadness, and trauma. Part III shares a method of health care for the general community, which you can offer your loved ones, or patients, if you are a healing professional of any kind.

The health issues we face today are real challenges, but with corrective rhythms therapy, we can regain spiritual, psychological, and physiological balance. These methods are well founded in clinical practices, yet this model requires our focus to shift from the illness model that has not served us well. The illness model thrives on our fears of pain and disease, in which degrees of healing are based on how many diseases we can control—not how healthy we can become to better defend ourselves against imbalances and invading illnesses. The end result is a continuous war against an unbeatable opponent because the world will always be a haven for organisms that compete against us for survival, even using our bodies as parasitic homes. To use a coaching metaphor, you don't encourage a kid to run a hundred-yard dash by making sure he doesn't fall or sabotage himself. No, you empower them to do their best. I want to empower you, and anyone you care for or treat, to be the best and healthiest person possible.

We'll know success when we are the healthiest nation we can be, instead of the least sick one. Through this book, I want to educate you on how that success can be attained and encourage you not to fear pain and disease. This is a curriculum for everyone to learn how to reset wellness based on the healing principles from history and learning to integrate with the universal powers that we are born with and have as our DNA. Our strong constitutions are the products of our ancestors; our health has been cultivating for thousands of years.

Our generation can boost those survival mechanisms with the discoveries that we now have.

This could be a breakthrough in health care, building on strengths instead of weakness and adding power to our DNA for future generations. That can be done, not by surgery or drug dependency, but by attitudes of promise and healthful behaviors. The quest for humanity is to grow into spiritual beings who reach our highest potentials. Achieving this feat can come through unifying the healing journey with rhythms of love and inner strength.

PART I

LIVING IN RHYTHM

A basic human drive is to find consistency in the moment so we can predict the future. That is the reason farmers needed intimate familiarity with the seasons, so they could plan and harvest their crops. Calendars were created to designate days of the year and loops around the sun. Scientists studied the stars at specific times to understand behavioral changes. Navigators also used the stars to guide their ships toward ports. Weather rhythms helped plan for the nurturance of sunshine and rain, and possible disasters. These measures are how we relate to the fluctuations of the universe and were imprinted on our DNA.

Just as there are fluctuations within the universe and our body rhythms, there are also rhythms of the planet and virtually all matter, even solid matter, through decay of energy and the vibrations of its particles. In essence, if we expand our sensitivities far enough, we will discover that all these rhythms fall into patterns. Within living beings, it is our nature that health persists through these universal patterns, and their disruption brings disharmony.

To maintain the order of rhythms and regulate humanity, rules were written to prevent the greed or immorality of human beings that disrupt everything. Wars have been fought over interpretations of events, and the end result is dismay at what we have done and defeat about human nature. The result of continuing imbalances are things as epic as climate change.

Being in harmony with natural rhythms means we are not resistant to change, rather we must adapt to it. Throughout the universe, there are needs for change. For example, black holes require changes in orbits of stars and planets to maintain balance. On an individual level, we must change behaviors to balance our metabolism according to our age and lifestyle. However, the kinds of changes needed and the power to make those changes are usually beyond human intellectual capacities and wisdom. Often, our major error as human beings is to over-control the rhythms of nature and thus create disasters. I would be very reluctant to have anyone try and regulate the tides of the oceans or the spin of the earth, yet we attempt medical interventions that do not account for natural balancing effects in our bodies.

The first part of this book is to bring awareness to a depth of appreciation for the importance of the rhythms that we encounter every hour of our lives. We begin with an exploration of how we might unify these powerful rhythms into an order which magnifies and directs that power toward health and wellness.

CHAPTER 1

HEALING RHYTHMS

I like to experience the universe as one harmonious whole. Every cell has life. Matter, too, has life; it is energy solidified. The tree outside is life.... The whole of nature is life.... The basic laws of the universe are simple, but because our senses are limited, we can't grasp them. There is a pattern in creation.
–Albert Einstein

When you're in pain or not feeling well, you likely take a pill or go to the doctor for medication that will make you feel better. It's no wonder, because drugs are the basis for our American medical system and they can be necessary. But does blindly following the Pill God and reaching for the latest wonder drug heal our whole being? Medications usually work fairly quickly, but there are many times when they don't.

Our healthcare system is the most expensive in the world, yet ranked only thirty-seventh among industrialized nations. Our lifespans, after centuries of increasing, now may be getting shorter. And it seems like the more effective and powerful our medicines become, the sicker we're getting. For every problem a medicine seems to solve, it creates a host of others. For example, lowering your cholesterol seems like a great idea, but the drugs you're using to help you do it may also be negatively affecting key body functions and brain activity. Cholesterol is a "brain food," and limiting or reducing it too much could be an invitation to insomnia. We alleviate the sleeplessness with medicines like Ambien and Lunesta, but those treatments have been linked to cognition issues, dementia—even Alzheimer's disease.

And what about pain? The opioids originally created and prescribed to treat significant pain from illness and injuries have become a full-blown addiction crisis that has claimed lives, shattered families, and threatens the US and world economies, as countless workforce hours are lost. The unscrupulous pharmaceutical industry and medical establishment have done little to address the crisis, often simply creating or prescribing another drug to replace the one before it.

We rush to medicate children—some as young as two years old—to "solve" attention and behavioral challenges, but the Ritalin- and Adderall-type drugs we give them may be interfering with their natural brain development. Many of these drugs are in the same class as cocaine and can become highly addictive, and their continued use can be devastating. Difficulty with anger management in relationships and in the workplace has been linked to childhood medical treatment of Attention Deficit Disorder (ADD) and Attention Deficit Hyperactive Disorder (ADHD) (Michelle M., 2017).

Perhaps most concerning, where does this global predicament leave us in our battles against diseases? Measles is back with a vengeance, historical threats like malaria and syphilis are rampant in parts of the world, and still others like the Zika and Ebola viruses continue to gather momentum.

We face some serious questions: Are we going forward or backward? On a merry-go-round of diagnoses leading to cures that create their own problems, which, in turn, require their own treatments, and so on, where does it end? Are we headed toward an Orwellian society in which we are all addicted to drugs that define our reality—and doom our country to eventual collapse? I like to think we will all learn better healing methods before that happens.

WHAT MEDICAL RESEARCH IS MISSING

Our approach to medical research may be at the heart of this threat. Treatments for illnesses, syndromes, pain, and anything else that ails us are usually developed using the "double-blind" approach, in which every possible variable is accounted for and controlled so that the effect of the drug in question can be isolated, quantified, and evaluated. The approach likely evolved from agricultural methods used to improve crop yields, and certainly has proven valuable in many scientific and medical applications. But double-blind research doesn't take into account how human healing happens.

Humans heal through what I call a "multiple-factor dynamic," because so much more is in play than one drug, a particular affliction, and just one part of the body. Simply put, we can't isolate and control all the variables. A person's attitude, emotional and mental states, metabolism, overall health, and many other factors influence the effects—positive and negative—of their illness or injury. It should also influence any treatments used. So using this "gold standard" of research, while it may look good on paper, is rather like trying to clear up a freeway traffic jam by checking the tire pressure of one car. What about all the other cars, and all their other parts? In the case of healing and wellness, environmental conditions, and how the parts of our bodies work together constitute the complexity of who we are, and ultimately, what keeps us healthy or makes us sick.

FEAR OF DISCOMFORT MAKES US SICKER

We don't die from things like pain. Often, our symptoms of illness or injury are helping us—even as they can cause us severe discomfort and force us to cease everyday functioning. We think we will die from them, but we likely won't. We're afraid of pain and illness, so we turn it into an enemy. But killing this enemy with medications and substances does not cure us; it just lulls us into a temporary comfort. This stops us from doing the things that do ease pain and illness, like stretching to break up scar tissue, doing gentle exercises to rebuild muscle, and sleeping in a way that rejuvenates the cells in our body. Over time, dependency on short-term treatments turns our body from friend to foe. In some cases, ever-increasing dosages bring side effects and an inability to interact with the world or fill our responsibilities to ourselves and our loved ones—much less to engage life full of joy and wonder.

This dependency feels like being caught in a web, where any string we pull damages some aspect of our life. Also, we do risk overdoses, botched surgeries, "just to be on the safe side" treatments, financial ruin from medical bills, and yes—we risk death. So when your doctor says you have reached the limit of a prescription and legally cannot give you any more, what will you do? Spend the rest of your life sick, in pain, and feeling despair? No. You can instead turn to innate healing rhythms. Many of these rhythms are within our individual bodies, but some of the most crucial ones are hidden within the secrets of the universe.

THE ROLE OF RHYTHMS WITHIN THE GALAXY

Even the dynamics of the heavens influence your health. Like many people, the word *universe* may get you thinking about outer space: planets, stars, and galaxies. You may picture illustrations of them. But the way we know these entities are out there is not visual—it's not like we can send video cameras so many millions of light years away to see these things. The giant telescopes that take readings of planets, stars, and galaxies do not provide visual images. They receive frequencies of energetic waves, which include sound waves. We track orbits and various behaviors of stars by the frequencies they exude. If you can convert those frequencies into musical notes, you would find that each planet and each star, and maybe even black holes, bring together a harmony of rhythm.

It's this rhythmic harmony that keeps the universe intact. It's a balance. The whole universe can be thought of as an orchestra. When it gets out of balance, it creates ways of re-balancing itself. It does that with the dark holes which swallow some energy, and we have explosions that go on in other parts of the universe. Try imagining all these parts of the universe as being like a composition.

Consider what Isaac Newton had to say on the idea. He described the universe as a clockwork of precision in which all the parts work with and pull against each other in perfect gravitational balance, much like our body systems work in concert with one another. Albert Einstein took the idea even further with the theory that the universe is constantly adjusting itself, or healing, to counteract constant, violent changes within it—like the births and deaths of planets, stars, and entire galaxies. Without these readjustments—these cosmic cures—our universe would likely collapse from the stress.

String theory shares an idea first put forth by Pythagoras that has become a vibrant field of study in modern physics. It suggests that the universe is a network of gravitational "strings." The strings vibrate at different frequencies, like instruments in an infinite celestial symphony, and maintain the order of the universe, much like your heartbeat regulates almost everything about you. To keep you healthy, your other systems revolve and respond to changes in stimuli, in a sort of biological give-and-take.

Our entire experience, as participants in this universe, is constantly changing. The awesome power and beauty of the music that shapes the change overwhelms our imagination. But it's also one of the keys to our health and happiness. The rhythms of the universe are felt in every aspect of our existence. Think about the creation stories of almost every culture, religion, and civilization; stories that explain and are based around seasons, celestial movements, tides, daylight and darkness, growing cycles, birth and aging and death. Our minds and bodies have evolved over the eons to work in concert with these cycles. We call these interdependent relationships our *circadian rhythms*, and they are the basis of our lives and our survival mechanisms. How well your rhythms function and respond to external challenges determines how well you adapt. In the big picture, those who adapt well will survive to reproduce, continuing and strengthening our species.

ANCIENT HEALING METHODS APPLY RHYTHMS

Cultures throughout the world, and for tens of thousands of years, have used rhythmic stimulation to harmonize and balance forces within the mind and body. According to Abd'el Hakim Awyan, an archaeologist and indigenous wisdom keeper in Egypt, the pyramids at Giza are harmonic structures designed to transmit the sound of flowing underground water. The reverberations were known to cure ailments by restoring a body's natural rhythms. Indeed, acoustician John Stuart Reid says his own chronic back pain was healed while he was conducting sound experiments within the chambers.

Possibly as far back as forty thousand years, Aborigines played the yidaki, similar to the didgeridoo, for healing purposes. Pythagoras taught flute and lyre as healing methods, and had his followers chant in unison to fight disease. The Greek Asklepion temples used music and imagery for attuning the body to its proper balance, and the collected ancient Greek texts known as *Corpus Hermeticum*, one of the earliest collections on physical and spiritual well-being, repeatedly reference music as a healing force.

Traditional Chinese medicine centers on balancing different energies in the body, and a primary diagnostic technique includes listening to the twenty-nine different pulses in our bodies. The qualities of this inner rhythm reveal how every organ in the body is functioning. And Ayurvedic medicine from India seeks the ideal balance between mind, body, and spirit by attuning activities and health treatments with the ways energy cycles every twenty-four hours.

To this day, many Native American medicine practitioners use songs, chants, drumming, and dancing as healing forces. These rituals are considered sacred information and confer special status on their practitioners. Instruments are created and receive special blessings for their power to promote healthy mental states. As part of my own recovery from a heart attack, I had the honor and privilege to participate in such a ritual, which used the songs of the bees to restore my natural rhythms.

Not only is dancing a fun physical activity, there is also evidence that virtually all ancient civilizations paired music with movement, whether in prayer for a successful hunt, a bountiful crop, victory in battle, or most notably, for healing and wellness. Dancing accentuates rhythm. As Einstein famously wrote, "Nothing happens until something moves," and, of course, one can hardly hear music without feeling the urge to dance. Since our whole universe, our entire lives, and our essential wellness are all rooted in fundamental rhythms, we are that much healthier when we move to the beat. And the best way to connect with these rhythms is in your own body.

THE POWER TO GROW BEYOND ANY IMBALANCE

I choose to empower people to be their own best sources of relief and healing. Rather than turning outside of yourself to ask doctors, healers, shamans—anyone at all—to fix you, consider taking responsibility and feeling power over your wellness. You *can* do healing things for yourself. I can offer you practices and activities, and you can gather your willpower, feel love for yourself, and do them. When you must expend as much, if not more, energy than any professional does to get better, this in itself is healing.

Learning skills for things you can do for yourself gives you power over illness, pain, and challenge. You have control, and you are no longer a victim of their nasty webs of effects and downward spirals. There is nothing like a taste of your own power to overcome the panic of not knowing what to do, find relief from imbalance, pull your life back together, and emerge stronger for having done it. Power will give you your life back and teach you to thrive amidst whatever life throws at you.

Throughout this book, I want to give you the tools you need, not pills or dependency of any kind. I want to give you access to your body, mind, spirit and show you the natural power to right any imbalance that is in your own being. As you journey through this book and do the exercises, you will make a fundamental shift in how you view your body. You will stop getting in its way, let its systems work, and augment its efforts by realigning with the inherent healing rhythms of balance in the universe.

This is a gentle and kind thing to do for yourself, which has incredibly profound implications for your well-being overall. I have watched thousands of people go through the process you are embarking on, and for each one, the journey evolves into a profound sense of spiritual connection. To be honest, you won't get far without it. So be at least a bit open to how spirituality will show up for you along the way—whether God's voice gets louder, you feel the warmth of love from above surrounding you, angels sing when you enter states of balance, you relax and let go into feeling grateful for what is, or you experience a kind of wonder that gives you access to feeling the greater flow of existence.

You have the potential to discover love for these rhythms that keep the universe's composition together. We experience this overriding melody as love. Each atom in our body has its own vibrations, and what keeps electrodes circling the nucleus is the attraction—the love—that is within itself. So draw the healing power of love to you by loving yourself, learning a new way of relating with wellness, and doing the practices in this book. Then, instead of being cut off from life, you will watch yourself return to the rhythms of its flow. Nothing is as beautiful and healing as that.

CHAPTER 2

THE BODY ORCHESTRA

Everything that exists in time has a rhythm and a pattern. Our bodies are multi-dimensional rhythm machines with everything pulsing in synchrony.
–Mickey Hart, percussionist and musicologist

We enjoy listening to a great orchestra perform largely because there is a sense of perfection. Everything is balanced. No sour notes. No clumsy rhythms. Everything is just right. We can surrender to the music and let it guide our mental and emotional experience. For a healthy body, timing and rhythm are also extraordinarily important factors. All our individual components are performing perfectly, together. Nature composed the music, our organs are finely tuned instruments, and everything is conducted by a maestro—our nervous system.

When we're healthy in body and mind, we just feel right. We're not simply getting through the day, we're enjoying it! The terrific feeling of well-being is taken for granted and we don't need to know the science behind it all; we just feel good, the way a great orchestra just sounds good. This harmonization of our body orchestra's frequencies is the blending together of different energies that naturally uplifts us, driving our spirit and passion for life.

When we are not healthy, our body orchestra is "out of tune," and the feeling that something's wrong nags us at most every turn. While anyone can listen to music and hear whether it sounds good or bad, and most people can sing or whistle a simple tune, it takes some music education to identify which of the many instruments in a symphony are hitting the sour notes. In the same way, when we're feeling poorly, it's tough to know which specific frequency is out of tune without some knowledge of our body's moving parts. In this chapter, I want to give you an overview of important physiological systems at work and also methods that return your personal body orchestra to harmony.

THE RESPONSIVENESS OF RHYTHMS

You can feel actual rhythms in your body. After all, what is your heartbeat if not a rhythm? All of your organs work on a rhythm, as do your hormones, regularly performing their functions as part of the biological orchestra that is you. That orchestra is a miracle of organization and interdependence, but it can also improvise. Our autonomic nervous system helps our bodies respond to danger, pain, illness, and stress in two fundamental ways.

First, there is the *sympathetic nervous system,* which reacts to a threat (say a tiger is after you) by triggering certain reactions: your senses are heightened, your pulse quickens to get more oxygen to your muscles so you can run away faster—and survive. Although the tiger example is extreme, it's an illustration of the body's desire and ability to take care of itself.

Once you've escaped the tiger, or the challenge to your everyday wellness, your *parasympathetic nervous system* encourages you to rest and relax to heal. While your sympathetic reactions help you fight off or escape threats, your parasympathetic system helps you heal and recuperate. You need this system to be healthy and functioning in order to repair injuries, conquer disease, and cope with the strains and stresses of daily life and survival.

Our parasympathetic system is incredibly powerful, but modern medicine largely ignores it. Sanitariums used to treat long-term illnesses by combining medical treatments with the activation of a patient's parasympathetic responses. While today's hospitals rarely engage this most potent healing approach, acknowledgment and integration of relaxation rhythms and parasympathetic responses go back to ancient times.

THE ELEVEN MAJOR ORGAN SYSTEMS

In any orchestra, there are four main sections: strings, woodwinds, brass, and percussion. Within those sections are a variety of instruments, from violins to trombones, and even those can have different parts to play in a composition. Similarly, your life is the result of eleven major organ systems that have many working parts.

Nervous system: the "conductor" of your body orchestra and the control center for everything that goes on inside you. Your brain, spinal cord, nerves, and all the organs that let you see, hear, feel, smell, taste, touch, and balance; they all receive and interpret stimuli and use that information to regulate all of your actions and reactions.

Cardiovascular (or circulatory) system: your heart and blood vessels, not to mention the blood that goes through them. This is the FedEx of your body, delivering the oxygen and nutrients your body "absolutely, positively" needs.

Respiratory system: using your mouth and nose, larynx and trachea, and lungs and diaphragm, you breathe in the oxygen that enriches the blood, and you breathe out carbon dioxide in the form of "used" air. Add sound and you're speaking—or singing.

Digestive system: the path your food and liquids take when you eat and drink, from your mouth down through your esophagus to your stomach and intestines. This system breaks down your food and extracts the nutrients and fuel your body needs.

Excretory system: processes and expels waste from your body when you go to the bathroom. Your kidneys, bladder, and colon are all key contributors.

Muscular system: supports and moves your body as muscle tissue tightens and relaxes. Ever seen athletes "warming up?" Feel hot after walking up a flight of stairs? Muscle movement generates heat.

Skeletal system: your bones and joints and all the connective tissue (like cartilage and tendons) between them. The skeletal system gives your body support and protects your internal organs. It also acts as a reservoir for important minerals like calcium, phosphorous, and magnesium.

Lymphatic system: the key to our natural immunity. It's a network of vessels and organs (including the spleen, tonsils, thymus gland, and lymph nodes) that form and transport lymphocytes, chemicals that fight off invasive cells.

Endocrine system: consisting of the pituitary, thyroid, and other glands, this system controls the creation and secretion of hormones that drive growth and development, regulate metabolism, and play a role in our moods.

Reproductive system: consisting of the organs (testes and ovaries) that produce sperm cells in males and egg cells in females; the sex organs; and the female uterus, where the fetus develops until birth.

Integumentary (skin) system: the skin system is so much more than just the bag you carry yourself around in. The skin system also includes your hair, nails, and the sweat glands that help you regulate body temperature and hydration, create vitamin D, and expel waste. Your skin is your first line of defense against infection, and as an anchor for sensory receptors it helps you detect pain, pressure, and temperature.

The core thing to perceive in this overview is that all these systems are interconnected. A problem in one system, even at the cellular level, can have far-reaching effects on our overall wellness. Illness in one organ is not an isolated event and treating it as if this were so, with pills, is not necessarily treating the problem. In my experience, the clinical reality of healing happens much differently.

I had a patient who was incredibly smart, but so out of touch with his body that he had severe high blood pressure, pain in his back, and problems with his vision. In our culture's medical system, he would be treated for three different things. Instead, I just taught him how to breathe in ways that engaged his parasympathetic nervous system so he could naturally rest and restore, connect to being embodied, and calm down in the midst of stress. With such a basic skill, he can see better, he feels better, his blood pressure is lower, and the pain has gone away. This philosophical shift, from mechanical and isolated parts to integrated whole-being systems, is a view that is at the heart of the wellness resets I discuss throughout this book.

MEASURING HEALTH WITH FREQUENCIES

The body orchestra is actually more than just an analogy about different parts working together to create something amazing. Your body and its different organs and systems actually create a sort of music. When you hear the different pitches in a tune (think "do-re-mi"), what's actually happening is that sound waves are vibrating at different frequencies—or the rates at which a vibration travels from one point to another. These frequencies are measured in Hertz or Hz (one Hertz means something is vibrating at one cycle per second), kilohertz or kHz, and megahertz or MHz (a megahertz is vibrating one million times per second). An orchestra's standard reference pitch is an "A" above "middle C," and it vibrates at 440 cycles per second, or 440 Hz.

Our organs and body systems have ideal frequencies too. You can't hear them, because the average human ear can't hear frequencies below 20 Hz (these are called infrasonic or subsonic frequencies) or above 20 kHz (called ultrasonic frequencies). In his book *The Body Electric*, Dr. Robert O. Becker wrote that a person's health could be ascertained by measuring the different frequencies the body produces. Later, the microbiologist and plant breeder Bruce Tainio built a machine called the BT3 to measure the frequencies of plants around the world. Several research organizations, including NASA, continue to pioneer new technology for measuring the frequencies of living things, including humans.

A healthy overall body frequency is generally thought to be in the 62 to 78 MHz range. (It usually slows down when you're sleeping.) A healthy brain frequency is between 72 and 90 MHz, and if you're in the upper half of that range, you might be a genius. The average heart vibrates at 68.5 MHz, lungs are in the 58 to 65 range, and so on.

It's in these numbers that the story of our health is told. As a cell's frequency starts to decrease, the cell stops functioning properly. If the frequency gets too low, below about 25 MHz, the cell can die. But well before that, a frequency drop of less than 10 MHz can make you vulnerable to a cold, flu, infection, and disease. A little more of a drop makes you more receptive to cancer. Frequency drops throw your systems out of balance with one another, and make your entire body have to work ever harder to carry out basic functions (Amit Sharma, 2017).

Even though your average doctor's office doesn't have a machine to measure your different frequencies and scientifically pinpoint the imbalances, we do have innate abilities to self-regulate our lives and promote our own health and wellness using methods that have been shown to bring physiological frequencies into balance.

METHODS TO SUPPORT OUR NATURAL HEALING RHYTHM ABILITIES

In 1937 the Nobel Laureate in Medicine, Albert Szent-Gyiorgyi, said that "In every culture and in every medical tradition before ours, healing was accomplished by moving energy." I call this innate blending and balancing of our body energies "natural healing rhythm abilities," and they are the key to keeping ourselves healthy. Every body instrument—nerve impulses, circulatory structures, organs, muscles, and more—must all work together to create *homeostasis*, a balanced harmony within the body. It's this majestic organization of countless tiny miracles that literally allows life. Even relatively minor breakdowns can have a surprisingly far-reaching effect, causing illness, disease, pain, and many other afflictions both physiological and psychological.

The frequencies and energy of the body do fluctuate in response to changes in stimuli and environment, and this is necessary and healthy, much the way a tree needs to bend in the wind so that it doesn't break. If you're happy, sad, afraid, surprised, angry, ashamed…all of those emotional states may cause adjustments in frequencies throughout your body to help you process your reactions. But on the whole, we need to keep our bodies in homeostasis, with our frequencies complementing one another, in order to be healthy.

What follows here are the practices I've found most helpful to my patients and instructive in my clinical research. These are natural arts—that is, they are so inherent in our nature that seldom are they subject to the "gold standard," the double-blind trials I mentioned in Chapter 1. So in laboratory parlance, they may not be considered "evidence-based." That said, I've been studying and deploying them for forty-five years, not to mention the thousands of years they've been informing the healing practices of cultures throughout the world. What better evidence is there than that?

The Art of Breathing

People often ask, "Why should I learn to breathe? I already know how." It's true, we breathe without even thinking about it. But if we *do* think about it and breathe consciously, we can adopt new, and variable, breathing patterns that complement our heartbeat and help us achieve optimal levels of energy, focus, relaxation, creativity, and more.

Try this: breathe *in* for 3 counts, *hold* it for 4 counts, then *exhale* for 5 counts. And again…3 in…4 hold…5 out. Again…3…4…5. You will instantly feel relaxed.

Scientists at the HeartMath Institute have researched and identified patterns using a device called the EmWave, which measures heart rate variability in response to different, deliberate breathing patterns. The controlled experiments and consistent results do, in fact, reach the standard of evidence-based methodology.

These conscious breathing patterns also influenced electro-encephalogram (EEG) readings, which identify brain activity. For example, as Dr. Barbara Peavey and I observed, the brain shows a heightened state of attention when subjects breathe in a "box" pattern: four counts in, four hold, four out, four hold, repeat. And the use of alternate-nostril breathing causes an upsurge in cross-hemisphere activity, usually manifesting as creative thinking.

I encourage you to experiment with the breathing exercises in this book. You will likely notice a shift in the way you feel. But even if you don't notice the change, your brain will. Breathing techniques have been used in the martial arts, music, meditation, and healing for a very long time. So while you don't have to learn how to breathe to "stay alive," the question is: Are you as alive as you could be?

Walking and Dancing

Walking is an integral part of your daily life. Sometimes you walk because you need to get somewhere, and other times, just for the pleasure of it. Dancing is usually either a romantic pastime or just for good old-fashioned fun, but it's also been used since the beginning of time in healing rituals and other aspects of spiritual life.

Both walking and dancing involve rhythm and balance. Even just shifting from one foot to the other requires communication within your brain. So movement is not just good for your body; it's also good for your brain. Without physical exercise, your brain hemispheres don't talk to each other enough, which can lead to depression. Movement releases dopamine and serotonin, which make you feel good. So every once in a while, or every day, get up, get down, and boogie! It will help lift your mood.

Moving in rhythm can help your body systems restore their own natural rhythms, coordinate into patterns with other systems, and harmonize your body orchestra. The result? Tension and stress start to melt away. If you've got a spouse or partner, dance with them! Dance is communication, so "listening to" another person's movements can foster better relationships.

Music Choices

It goes without saying that just about everybody loves music. Think of the billions of dollars spent on recordings, concert tickets, musical instruments, and lessons. And think how just about every holiday or special occasion we celebrate has at least some songs or pieces identified with it. Why do we love music? Because it stimulates our brains in so many ways. When you hear a song, you're actually hearing multiple characteristics at once, and they each affect your brain in a unique way.

Tempo is the speed or pace of the music and it makes you want to move, if not by dancing, then at least by snapping your fingers or tapping your toes. Slow tempos make you feel calm, either in a serene, peaceful sense or in a contemplative or sad way. Quicker tempos excite you, making you exuberant, or angry, or alert.

Mode is the type of musical scale used in a song or piece. "Do-re-mi," the song from *The Sound of Music*, is based on a "major" scale, and it has a happy, joyous, celebratory feel. "Minor" scales have a more somber feel and are often used to convey a sad feeling. "Someone Like You" by Adele is a good example.

Loudness, or what we often call volume, is simply how loud or soft a piece of music is. Louder music tends to give us more of a feeling of intensity (good or bad), while quiet music might make us more thoughtful.

Melody is the arrangement of pitches in a scale into what we call "the tune." Along with complementary harmonies (that guy who shows off singing the last line of "Happy Birthday" differently from everyone else), the melody is perhaps most responsible for the feel of a song or piece.

If music inspires us to move *and* creates responses in our brains (not to mention our hearts and souls), it's a miraculous thing indeed. The connection between music, movement, and the brain was illustrated perfectly by a story on the *Ellen* show. A young man with severe autism also lived with severely impaired motor control that made him unable to perform more subtle movements. He had always dreamed of working as a server at Starbucks, but his limitations made that chance slim, at best. That's when fate stepped in. A man with a knowledge of music and a relationship with Starbucks took an interest in the young man, helping him integrate his serving movements with carefully selected musical selections. Sure enough, through his own intense effort, he got the job of his dreams.

For millennia, music has bridged the gulf between despair and hope, suffering and healing, in cultures around the world.

Throughout my career, I've researched the connection between music and wellness, and recommended specific music to patients and friends alike. Along with colleagues Mark Rider and Jeanne Achterberg, I published an article on the positive effects of music on the immune system (Rider, 1989).

The only limitation I faced—and it was a giant one—was the process of selecting music uniquely suited to each person. I knew the types of frequencies and rhythms these folks needed, but finding the right music each time was a needle-in-a-haystack proposition. So I started creating my own music for my patients. Now lest you think I'm the next Beethoven, rest assured that my music is very simple, based entirely on rhythms and sounds targeted to specific desired brain responses. Try them for yourself—my music is downloadable from www.mindbodybylawlis.com.

Yoga and Tai Chi

Both of these ancient arts combine breathing with movement to help you stay relaxed and focused. Yoga teaches "equanimity amidst intensity," or the ability to deflect stress more easily and completely. The breathing component of these ancient arts engages your parasympathetic nervous system, the branch that manages how you respond to stressors. Plus, the movements help your brain hemispheres communicate. Mind-body exercises that activate your parasympathetic nervous system are terrific for your endocrine and immune systems, improving your overall health and body function in addition to their positive effect on your stress levels. Mind-body techniques have proven so effective that National Health Interview Surveys from 2002 to 2012 ranked tai chi, yoga, and qigong as the most popular complementary health approaches in America (Wang, 2017). All three combine movement, breathing, and focus.

Tai Chi combines martial arts movements with the elements of *Qi*—your vital energy, circulation, breathing, and stretching. The movements, performed while standing, are slow and graceful, the breathing deep and from the diaphragm.

Yoga combines muscular activity (movement and stretching) with mindful focus on self-awareness, breathing, and energy. With yoga, you can integrate your physical, mental, and spiritual self to reduce stress and achieve greater wellness.

Qigong is a series of breathing practices combined with body movement and meditation. Through qigong, you cultivate the vital energy in your body to achieve a state of deep focus and relaxation.

All three of these arts involve every facet of your being. Their universal theme is that everything within you and about you is always connected, so you must always pay attention to the whole you. These ancient practices developed over centuries of refinement, and they function almost like a tuning fork for your body.

Healing Touch

There is tremendous healing power in human touch. In some ways, its power doesn't need to be explained—we use it every day. My mother, a schoolteacher, used simple touch when she had a difficult, angry student. All she had to do was touch their arm and that anger would dissipate. I came to appreciate its use in healing during a workshop, and I invited a practitioner to come to my pain clinic and demonstrate just what this "laying on of hands" could do for patients.

The clinic had one man who had been hit by a crane and was in excruciating pain. He spent every moment he was awake crying out for pain medication that would just put him to sleep, knock him out, so he couldn't feel anything at all. He lived with nothing in between. I suggested that the energy worker go to his room and see if he could do anything for the man's pain.

After about thirty minutes, I noticed that the man wasn't yelling anymore. Then ten minutes after that, I saw the patient dancing down the hall. He was singing, over and over again, "I'm cool. I'm good. I'm great!" I thought that was fascinating, so I sent the energy worker to another patient. I set my stopwatch and, forty minutes later, the patient came out dancing. He treated four more patients and, every time, in forty minutes they were dancing.

I thought this talent might be unique to the practitioner, but he insisted that he could show anyone how to do it. So I hired him to teach me and the entire staff. We used his method and it worked tremendously well.

Many healing modalities embrace the power of healing touch. There is Reiki, a discipline called Shen, acupressure, and of course massage. In the 1970s, the pioneering nurse Dolores Krieger, PhD, began a series of experiments on what she called Therapeutic Touch. The findings were so significant that there are now more than one hundred thousand Therapeutic Touch practitioners within all walks of medicine. Similarly, many nurses have become certified in the Healing Touch method. In some sense, we can all be healers through touch. Yet being trained in knowing how to touch another human being and transfer healing energy has been shown to have tremendous effects on health.

Aromas

The relationship between your brain and certain aromas is amazing. Do aromas have frequencies? Maybe not, but regardless, they do have a powerful effect on your response to stress. Inhaling certain aromas can serve as a snap-out-of-it slap in the face that brings your focus back to reality from exaggerated levels of worry and anxiety. It's not an escape so much as a reset to your normal, healthy brain frequency.

Why is aroma such a powerful and immediate influence on our brains? It might be because our olfactory nerve centers are very close to the brain, or that, over the eons, our sense of smell developed as part of the attention mechanism that helps us survive. Our reaction to an aroma travels quickly to the limbic system in the brain, which is partially responsible, not only for some body functions, but for our emotions as well.

Solitude

Humans are social animals; society expects us to congregate, play a role in our community, have friends, seek companionship, and receive professional help when we're feeling poorly. If we don't build and exercise these relationships every day, it seems, we're seen as antisocial hermits who "need help." We may even be branded "borderline personalities" or "sociopaths."

To be sure, contact, warmth, love, reassurance, and support are all critical to your wellness, and a life completely devoid of other people and interactions is surely lacking. But… sometimes you just need to be alone. Despite psychologists, practitioners, and friends who want to be desperately needed all the time, there comes a time in any healing process—physical, mental, or emotional—when you'll need time to process, practice, succeed and fail, and learn to "stand on your own two feet" again.

Think about some of the challenges you face, right now, to your own well-being. Do any of them involve stress at work or in your family? Are you "unpacking" issues, past or present, that stem from your own childhood? Your marriage? Your own children? Your job? On one hand, it's great to have someone to help you through. But on the other, it sounds like you're already hosting quite a crowd in your head, with each person's voice, opinion, personality, and role in the matter vying for your attention.

Ultimately, balance and harmony comes from inside *you*. In many cultures, a young person embarks on a Vision Quest, a personal journey of self-discovery. They set off in solitude in search of a truth that only they can discover. Who they will be or what role they will play in society is not dictated to them by an authority figure or any societal demand or expectation. Ancient traditions and stories tell of these journeys, beset with challenges that, in the end, reveal the seeker's path and purpose. Do you need to fast in the desert for forty days and nights, like Jesus, to work through your challenges and find balance in your life? No, but make sure solitude has space and time in your healing regimen.

If you've ever lost a loved one, hopefully you've had caring people to console and support you. But after a while, their attention might begin to feel like its own burden, leaving you exhausted and desperate for time alone with your thoughts. It's in that solitude that you'll begin to find your balance and a sense of normalcy, and finally begin to just be *you* again.

Our brains are actually way ahead of us on this idea. In solitude, we are often able to visualize an ideal state, free of challenge, danger, and fear. It's not that those challenges don't exist, it's that we are able to shift our focus to the goal; we reframe the problem and set our eyes on the prize. If you could see your brain as this shift happens, you'd see an almost immediate change in frequency as your brain restores itself to its healthy rhythm.

As a psychologist, I have to admit that it's taken some time and humility on my part to realize that my direct involvement in a patient's care is not the be-all and end-all, and that the most crucial elements in healing and wellness come with self-discovery. We can harness activities that support our innate ability to heal, and integrate them into our lives and treatment practices. If pharmacy and surgery could be seen as components of the whole healing process—and not the be-all end-all—that would be the most exciting thing in the world to me.

We can do this. The whole-being methods of treatment shared in this chapter draw from history and ancient medicine in experientially and clinically tested applications. They broadly apply what works to harness our healing forces in concentrated ways. In the next chapter, I'll extend that idea to share how you can transform your life through your natural healing rhythms by gaining freedom from destructive brain patterns and integrating new opportunity, behaviors, and beliefs into your life.

CHAPTER 3

BRAIN TOOLS FOR CHANGE

I know of no more encouraging fact than the unquestionable
ability of man to elevate his life by conscious endeavor.
–Henry David Thoreau

Your brain truly is an amazing organ. Just when we think we know everything about how the brain works, new theories arise, new discoveries are made, and we wonder all over again if we'll ever fully understand these most powerful and mysterious little supercomputers that live inside our skulls. What is it that keeps us from being just a race of identical robots, devoid of any critical thinking skills or individuality? Maybe there's something magical happening, but there's also a lot of biology, chemistry, and physics that we can work with to keep the brain in tune and the body firing on all cylinders.

Our brain naturally changes throughout our lifetime, which gives us the ability to heal mentally and emotionally by changing our brain's physiology. This ability is widely embraced as *neuroplasticity*. So just as our brain gets affected by imbalances and illnesses, we can reset it by learning and repeating healing neural pathways. In this chapter, I'll share work I've done to analyze and stimulate different parts of the brain in different ways, the results my patients have seen, and how you can treat your own brain better.

THE BRAIN MAP

Viewed from the side, our brain appears to be divided into five major parts, or lobes. Each lobe manages particular brain functions.

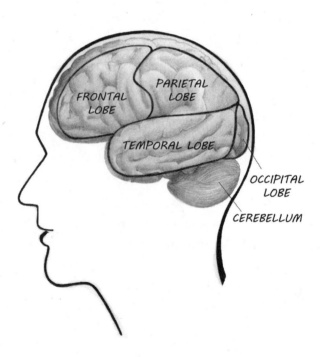

FRONTAL LOBE

PARIETAL LOBE

TEMPORAL LOBE

OCCIPITAL LOBE

CEREBELLUM

The *frontal lobe* controls memory, organization, planning, and impulse control. When this lobe is injured, a person may be scattered, easily angered or frustrated, and unable to recall even basic information.

Behind the frontal is the *parietal lobe*, the logical processing region of the brain. It helps you understand language, concept formation, cause-and-effect relationships, and more. Damage to this area might affect your ability to see or make conclusions and solve puzzles and problems.

The *occipital lobe*, at the very back of the brain, transforms the light gathered by your eyes into the information you "see." A damaged occipital lobe can cause blindness or hallucinations.

In front of the occipital, near the temples, is the *temporal lobe* which not only processes your emotions, but helps you understand others' emotions as well. The temporal lobe also plays critical roles in language and information processing. Injury in this area may impact levels of empathy and comprehension.

The fifth lobe, perched right atop your spinal cord, is called the *cerebellum*. This lobe controls your coordination and movement. You might suspect trouble in this lobe if you suddenly had trouble walking or performing basic physical tasks.

These five lobes, as you may have already guessed, do not operate in isolation. The functions and health of one lobe will significantly affect the other lobes and brain function as a whole.

Here's an example. You're in the attic, searching for that old rock concert t-shirt in a pile of forgotten clothes, when suddenly you hear (temporal lobe) a rattling sound from underneath the pile. Your brain quickly searches in your memory (frontal lobe) for the meaning (parietal lobe) of that auditory signal. It's a rattlesnake! You catch a glimpse (occipital lobe) of the critter slithering under an old coat, and if you were raised in west Texas, you might even recognize its smell (deep regions of the parietal lobe). Your frontal lobe starts forming an escape plan, and your cerebellum cranks up your arms and legs so you can, well, get the hell out of there. That's a pretty complex operation, and if any part of the sequence doesn't play out, you're in for a rough afternoon.

Now that you've seen your brain in action, let's look at your brain from the top. There's a division right down the middle between the two sides, or *hemispheres*. Since many nerves crisscross in your brain, the *left* hemisphere exerts the most control over the *right* side of your body, and vice-versa. Also, the left hemisphere is commonly thought to be more rational, logical, and analytical, while the right side is more emotional, empathetic, and creative.

Encasing the whole thing is an outer layer called the *cerebral cortex*, or simply cortex. It's the electrical impulses in the cortex that are picked up and measured when you get an electroencephalogram, or EEG. The frequencies of these charges are categorized by the level of information being processed in different areas of the cortex.

- At the Delta level (0.5–4 Hz), little or no data is being processed. You're asleep.

- At the Theta level (4–8 Hz), you're in a hypnogogic state, the transition between being awake and asleep.

- Alpha level (8–12 Hz) means you're awake, but you and your brain are relaxed. Not a lot of data being processed.

- The Beta level (12–15 Hz) is your optimal data processing level. You're alert, focused, and learning. But if you get to a High Beta level (16 Hz or higher), you're in data overload. There's a lot of information, but you're not processing it efficiently. You're stressed and anxious.

When we measure brain activity, we can see if there's consistency from the different regions, which in most cases, would be a good thing. For example, if we get a Beta measurement from all over the cortex, we know your brain as a whole is in good shape for learning. But conflicting levels of activity from one region to the next mean your brain is being counterproductive. The good news is we've learned how to harmonize those frequencies, optimizing whatever your brain needs to do in a particular situation: learn, move, rest, sleep, and more.

HEALING YOUR BRAIN THROUGH FREQUENCIES

Over the years, I've learned that my sophisticated training in traditional talk therapy does not always help my patients as advertised. While that can be a blow to my ego, it's also the impetus to explore and develop new treatment methods. As I started to study and learn more about frequencies and rhythms, I began to incorporate drumming into my therapy. It was immediately beneficial to many patients, but I learned the hard way that not everyone in nearby departments—even on other floors—appreciates the sound of drumming during the workday. There had to be another way.

I turned to my son, whose knowledge of electronic engineering helped us develop a device to deliver frequencies, controllable and variable by the patient, to each ear. As a patient, you control the pitch you're hearing in each ear by turning the frequency knobs. There are also knobs for volume. As you experiment, you begin to notice changes in your symptoms, mental and emotional states, and overall sense of wellbeing. I fine-tuned this process and created the Bio-Acoustical Utilization Device (BAUD).

This type of interaction between technology and a patient's self-regulation of symptoms is known as *biofeedback*, a clinical designation important in classifying diagnosis and treatment. In our trials, we observed and recorded significant repeatable improvements using the BAUD, meeting every standard for evidence-based treatment. The device has since received FDA approval for use in biofeedback-based treatment. Because I'm one of the inventors of the device, I can't publish my own results in peer-reviewed publications, where the appearance of conflict of interest must be avoided. Nevertheless, many rehabilitation programs throughout the world have adopted the BAUD, and the Navy SEALs are considering possible applications as well.

A powerful reason why BAUD therapy works is that it addresses a significant structure in our brain, called the *amygdala*. A lot of people are talking about the amygdala now because it is the recorder of negative emotions. I've written extensively about how the amygdala is highly sensitive to music and to rhythms (Lawlis, 2008). Brain frequencies born out of a trauma—such as a surgery, accident, or other physically or emotionally harming event—need to be stopped and disrupted. For example, with post-traumatic stress disorder (PTSD), we can find the frequency that's causing anxiety and disrupt it with sound in order to replace it with a more curative rhythm. Sound has been shown to directly affect the amygdala to arouse the memories stored there, fine-tune them so they can be resolved, and create new ways of responding physiologically that enhance well-being, instead of upset and suffering (Miller, 2017).

This can be very helpful for managing the emotional responses to illness, something that is essential to do because negative emotions have physiological effects that make any sickness worse. Research has shown the BAUD to be incredibly effective because it enhances a neural reset that reduces or eliminates symptoms. We've used the BAUD for a multitude of applications, and are most impressed with results in pain reduction and the stimulation of brain activity. And over the years, with more than four thousand cases, there has never been a negative side effect caused by the BAUD. Not one.

RESTORE YOUR BRAIN THROUGH SENSORY DEPRIVATION

Sometimes the key to finding balance and restoring rhythms requires shutting out as much of the world around us as possible. In my practice, I've often included sensory deprivation to help peel away layers of distraction, stress, conscious thought, and extraneous stimuli so that a patient's brain is essentially forced into a relaxed, parasympathetic, healing and restorative state. It's an exceptionally powerful mechanism that naturally eases our brain into the Theta level frequency, and works even better when combined with other therapies like breathing and sound. Patients who have spent time in isolation therapy have reported episodes of extraordinary clarity, spiritual awakening, and even a sense of a divine presence in their lives much more profound than what they might experience in a house of worship or in traditional prayer.

I often send patients in larger metropolitan cities to spas that offer "float therapy," where you can indulge in a zero-gravity experience of floating in water with a thousand pounds of Epsom Salt dissolved into it. You can also create your own sensory-deprivation chamber, and I have built them, but to tell the truth, even in a clinic or hospital setting, it can be problematic, labor-intensive, potentially expensive, and sometimes just not practical or possible. It's easy enough to create darkness and control or prevent physical activity, but the infiltration of sound is harder to eliminate. Still, sensory isolation is valuable, so to the extent that you can create your own simplified deprivation environment, you should give it a try. Even a setup as basic as a mattress or yoga mat on the floor of a dark closet, wearing a sleep mask and good earplugs, may help you approximate the experience to some degree. Deepen your experience by using the breathing patterns described in this book or by listening to some healing music.

RESET YOUR BRAIN WITH MUSICAL SOUNDS

If someone mentions Beethoven's Fifth Symphony, you think first and foremost about *dun-dun-dun-duuuuun*, or the opening melodic line. But that's just our conscious mind reacting. While melodies like this—or the tunes we sing along to—may be what we use to identify a piece of music, our bodies react the most to rhythm. You tap your toes to it. You bounce in your chair to it. You drum on your steering wheel to it (carefully!), and of course, you dance to it. Different rhythms can drive feelings of energy and power, spirituality, and romance. Dr. Mark Rider and I even identified certain rhythms, such as marches, that influence group dynamics (Mark S. Rider, 1989).

The sound-stimulation compositions I've created are based on physiological and brain changes I've observed through years of monitoring responses to different frequencies and rhythms. There was a lot of trial and error, a lot of material in the trash bin, and a lot of music that wouldn't necessarily fit anyone's personal definition of the word. (At times, I thought my recording studio engineer might explode in frustration.)

Forget about the three-and-a-half-minute pop songs created to meet radio-industry demands (and much earlier, the space limits of 78-rpm records). Using modern looping technology, we've created compositions that are several hours long. The recordings available for downloading at www.mindbodybylawlis.com are timed for maximum effect. Here are some of the compositions that reset your brain and can therefore change your life.

Joy and Peace: This CD was constructed and performed at my house by four clinic staff members. It's about twenty-two minutes of drumming and rhythms based on the Theta frequency, which occurs during the hypnagogic state between wakefulness and sleep. Our original intent was to promote the dreamlike imagery that often accompanies that state, but many of our subjects reported feelings of positivity and optimism. Their brain frequencies increased to Alpha and Beta levels, moods lifted from their previous depressive levels, and they performed physical and cognitive tasks better.

Homeostasis: I created a composition by combining the frequencies associated with the harmonic relationships between the body's eleven systems (described in Chapter 2) when they are in homeostasis with one another. I included an underlying rhythm based on the Alpha frequency. The physiological reactions, such as heart rate, breathing, and galvanic skin response (GSR), most often indicated relaxation, as I had expected. Subjects' verbal responses varied but were positive and included observations such as, *"I felt my chakras line up."* Many folks use this particular recording in the morning to organize their energies for the day, while others use it to relax.

Entropy: Why is it so hard sometimes to fall asleep and stay asleep? You need sleep to allow your brain and body to recuperate from all the hard work they do during the day, and yet those Delta frequencies can be so elusive. Your brain has to "trust itself" to let go of its normal level of activity and leave itself open. So I created a sound pattern to help get you there. In my practice, I often use this recording as a complement to the sensory deprivation chamber. The vulnerability of an open mind leads to highly emotional but very positive responses.

Awakening: Sometimes the frequencies traveling between your brain's hemispheres or among its different lobes are skewed, which can correlate with depression and drug dependency. The rhythmic pattern I developed to combat those discrepancies directs different frequencies to your right and left ears at different times, mimicking and complementing the pattern of alternate-nostril breathing (which you should try as you listen). The treatment helps first to "recharge" the individual lobes and separate hemispheres. Then as the different sounds come together in both ears, the different brain areas are brought together in concert.

Gonging: The deep, lasting ring of a gong is powerful and relaxing, and a great groundwork for addressing attention issues like ADD, ADHD, and even OCD. Along with occasional verbal reminders over the steady gonging, the recording helps you strengthen your own ability to stay focused and on-task amidst a sense of calm. You might recognize similarities between this type of brain training and meditation strategies that focus on breathing and movement. The steady gong sound can accentuate the power of meditation by reinforcing consistent rhythm. Even after just three to five minutes, the change in your mental state feels empowering. And as with each of these sound programs, the more you use it the better it works.

The Heart Frequency: Perhaps the most powerful of all the body's frequencies in addressing pain and stress is the frequency of the human heartbeat. I've witnessed that power in an incredibly diverse range of settings— from the drumming at Native American conferences and meetings to the comfort children received from their mother's heartbeat in a pediatric burn ward, where no medication in the world can alleviate the pain of daily skin debridement. Neither medications nor alcohol can take the place of nature's rhythms in helping you through stress, pain, and the several stages of sleep. Only the frequency of the heartbeat can do that. That's how—and why—this recording works.

Stable States: Our brains can be destabilized by trauma or drugs to the point that we are unable to understand communication and experience confusion with even simple logics. When you're in this state, you might feel you're in a world where nothing makes sense anymore. When anyone tries to tell you something that could be meaningful and useful in your life, the message gets lost in translation or decoding. The music that helps with this consists of a complex chord with a silent beat in which the mind hears slight differences in the combination of sounds. Through self-restructuring, you gain a sense of clarity.

FOOD THERAPY FOR YOUR BRAIN

You've heard it all your life: eat right. We know that food choices affect heart health, organ function, and ultimately your lifespan. But the wrong foods also are a sure ticket to dysregulation of your natural rhythms. You'll just feel off: tired, cranky, stressed, unfocused, frustrated. Who wants that?

Simply put, food is medicine. And natural foods are the best natural medicine. But in recent decades, ever-growing demands on the world's food supply—and the ever-accelerating quest for profits by corporate megaproducers—has led to the use of science and technology to increase quantity at the expense of quality. Genetic engineering, hormones, antibiotics, pesticides, and our insatiable addiction to sugar have all taken a toll on our health and wellbeing.

The good news is, if you know which foods are the good guys and which are the bad, you can make choices that complement and strengthen the natural rhythms of your organs (especially your brain), bolster your immune system, and contribute to a longer, more vibrant life. This basic level of health can do wonders for your emotions and spirit.

The biggest villain in our food story is processed sugar. Unlike many food ingredients, such as fats, where we take the pros with the cons, added sugars offer zero benefit to our health. All they do is add calories, rot your teeth, and interfere with critical organ functions. Sugar is a major factor in diabetes, liver complications, skin problems, obesity, stress, immunity decline, cardiac issues, cancer…the list goes on. And because it triggers pleasure-producing neurotransmitters, sugar can be dangerously addictive. Sugar substitutes can be just as bad or worse, essentially acting as toxins in your brain and body. Among other problems, long-term use of some substitutes can lead to cognitive decline.

The other bad guys taking over your grocery store are chemical food preservatives and insecticides. Your body simply does not know what to do with these substances, so they linger in your organs as toxins, causing inflammation in your body and in your brain, where they wreak havoc on your metabolism and create imbalance in your immune responses.

To get these bad actors out of your life, try to find and buy organic and non-genetically modified produce and meats. They're a little more expensive, but your well-being is worth it. (They taste better, too.) And although I couldn't possible name every food you're better off skipping, here are a few examples you should leave on the store shelf.

- Beer and mixed drinks (sorry!)

- Simple carbohydrate foods like most breads, rolls, biscuits, and bagels

- Starchy vegetables like corn and peas

- High-carb fruits like bananas, raisins, mangos, and those without skins or leaves

- Processed foods like French fries, soda, potato chips, limiting anything that comes in a box or can

- Deep-fried and battered foods

- Candy, cakes, pastries, and anything containing processed sugar.

After seeing some of your favorite foods on that list, take heart! The list of foods you should eat for a healthy brain and body, well-tuned rhythms, better immunity, and powerful energy is much longer, and I've only scratched the surface. You're about to be hungry....

Pack in the protein: beef, from burgers to steaks to prime rib to the holiday roast; chicken and duck; tuna, salmon, trout, halibut, any fish you can "reel in"; shrimp, crab, lobster (and, yes, you can have the melted butter too), cheeses, salami, pastrami, sausages, ribs (watch out for the sauce), buffalo wings, liverwurst, oysters, abalone, a variety of nuts, protein powders.

Like Mother always said, eat your veggies: broccoli, spinach, lettuce, cabbage, bok choy, kale, asparagus, mustard greens, mushrooms, cucumbers, pickles, celery, green beans, Brussels sprouts, cauliflower, artichokes, peppers, onions, sprouts (bean, alfalfa, etc.), radicchio and endive, herbs like parsley, cilantro, basil, rosemary, thyme; radishes, sea vegetables, jicama, avocado, asparagus, green beans and wax beans, summer squash, zucchini, scallions or green onions, bamboo shoots, leeks, snow peas (pods), tomatoes, eggplant, tomatillos, artichokes, fennel, okra, spaghetti squash, celery root (celeriac), turnip, water chestnuts, pumpkin, nuts, flaxseeds.

Fruits offer terrific antioxidants: grapefruit, lemons, limes, strawberries, olives, raspberries, blackberries, kiwis, plums, oranges, pears, pineapple.

Oils, mustard, salt, pepper, soy sauce, tea, coffee, cream, sugar-free Jell-O, some salad dressings, and the occasional glass of wine (a toast to your good health!) are okay too.

Do you have allergies or sensitivities to certain foods? A food that's on the "good" list is not necessarily right for *you*. As you design your diet, you may uncover more foods that, in one way or another, make you uncomfortable or cause problems. Keep a food diary that tracks what you eat, when you eat it, and how your body, mind, and mood react to it. You'll soon have a healthy, tasty diet that keeps your brain in balance and feeling great.

All these methods are geared to boost your brain function, so it can adapt to change and coordinate the healthy function of all your body's systems. Change is a basic fact in our universe. When it happens in stars and galaxies, and throughout the year on earth as the seasons rotate, we cannot expect that we will defy this principle and stay the same. As life goes on, the conditions inside and outside us require that we change too, so resisting it is futile and self-harming.

The best relationship to change that you can have is to regard it as good news. Whatever issue you may be facing in your life, it will change—guaranteed. You can even set its direction through intentional actions and behaviors. The next part of this book gives you specific ideas for integrating what you've learned so far into your everyday life so you can promote healthier body rhythms and recover balance in your life. A basic tempo of well-being affects everything.

PART II

HEALING CORE IMBALANCES

With an understanding that the rhythms of human beings can be shifted to healthier states through the utilization of sounds, movements, and brain patterns, now pretend you are a fly on the wall, watching and observing stories of people whose normalcy in rhythmic life was disrupted by conflict or trauma. These are stories of healing in which there is not one singular answer, cure, or quick fix for their imbalance and a combination of approaches proved successful. Most importantly, the love and understanding that accompanied their treatments served to reset a basic sense of safety and possibility.

Throughout our lives, we each encounter many instances of rhythmic disruption, as each chapter of life brings challenges to confront us and help us grow. It would take many volumes to detail one life, full of transitions, and consider the many approaches that can facilitate successful healing. This book is not meant to be a panacea or *the* answer to all of life's problems.

Rather, it's intended to reveal to you the power behind the rhythms you can reset for wellness.

Consider Part II a guide to common opportunities for rhythmic reset that have shown tremendous ability to change lives, from states of suffering to health and well-being. I portray the horrors of insomnia, pain, depression, and trauma to demonstrate that change is possible at any stage of life, within the challenges of any disease, and beyond the fracture of one's passion or love.

CHAPTER 4

SLEEPING IN A CIRCADIAN RHYTHM

*Even a soul submerged in sleep is hard at work and
helps make something of the world.*
–Heraclitus

The most basic rhythm for life on earth is day and night. Our entire world and every creature in it move in sync with the cycle of transitioning from light to dark, and then to light again. We each experience this twenty-four-hour clock, known as a *circadian rhythm,* as the stunning oranges, pinks, and purples of sunrises and sunsets, which cue us to head outdoors or indoors and, most essentially, to prepare to awaken or to sleep.

I associate sunsets with running toward home as a boy, the sky darkening around me late on summer nights, my legs tired from a day of playing football or riding bikes. I knew that, soon, I would be told to wash up and brush my teeth, climb into bed with a book, be kissed goodnight, and the lights would go out. Rituals like this are part of us, from childhood until the end of our lives, because as night falls, people across earth turn to the comfort of our beds to rest up for the next day.

This is a natural and innate part of being human, as is waking to the sun and rising for another cycle of activity. It is so inherent that sometimes we can take it for granted, forget its value, and fall out of the healing cycle of sleep's regeneration. The hardships and trauma we experience in life can cause us to become too distressed or fearful to fall asleep. We can become overly stimulated by activities, not bother transitioning into a relaxed state, or struggle to let go of our rational and problem-solving minds in order to surrender to a dream state. These are all ways we fall out of sync with our natural circadian rhythm.

Every single person alive would agree, based on experience, that no one can function long without sleep. We all have times when we struggle with insomnia, whether there's a new baby or puppy crying through the night, we're feeling overwhelmed by a task we face, there's a problem we get obsessed with solving, or we're too emotional to stop rehashing events. Of all the people who come to me for help, for whatever issue, I'd say 75 percent have also developed sleep problems. We each get this rhythm thrust out of balance for all kinds of reasons. But unless we resolve sleep issues, all other healing is prevented. One of the secrets to harnessing our healing rhythms for a life of wellness is returning our sleep to nature's circadian clock.

WHEN SLEEP IS DISRUPTED, WE FALL APART ON ALL LEVELS

I was looking out my office window one day, watching as gusts of strong Texas wind repeatedly pushed a woman off course as she tried to make it to the door. I knew this must be Pere (pronounced like *Perry*), who wanted help with insomnia. I was worried that, small as she was and skinny as a rail, she might be blown away with the wind. When she arrived, she was very tense around her shoulders, as if carrying a thousand-pound load. Her eyes darted around the room, not wanting to focus, and her whole being seemed stressed out by the basics of daily demands. She hardly spoke louder than a whisper, as if she might awaken a giant demon if she talked too loudly.

It was clear that Pere's overall physical and psychological health was suffering from her inability to sleep and enter a parasympathetic state to rest and restore. The mechanics within the rhythm of alternating between sympathetic and parasympathetic states are controlled primarily through the brain by the *hypothalamus,* which is light sensitive. This regulates the release of *melatonin,* which is a hormone that regulates the sleep-wake cycle (among other things). The secretion of these hormones is related to the sensation of light and dark, which goes back to the beginning of humankind and the beginning of life itself. We need to respect this cycle of activity and rest, as interruptions in the rhythm can cause emotional, hormonal, and genetic disorders. The usual symptoms are anxiety, depression, lack of attention, fatigue, poor focus, impulsivity, damaged interpersonal relationship, and poor job performance—just to name a few.

Pere was experiencing enough of these symptoms to have become obsessed with her inability to sleep. It is common, and you likely do this during periods of insomnia, to create rituals like not drinking coffee, not eating spicy food at dinner, making teas, taking a bath, and even ignoring or avoiding inter-actions with other people that might make you feel stressed. The belief is that this ongoing ritual is going to guarantee sleep that night. This is a form of performance anxiety, which professional musicians and athletes also experience. For example, a baseball player may rub a bat ninety-eight times in one direction and forty-three times in the other direction.

Pere's rituals had become so extreme that they began governing her day at one o'clock in the afternoon. She even refused to have conversations with people—with the remote possibility of making her upset—after three o'clock. Pere reported the anger she felt toward others when they intruded on her various schemes. Turns out Pere had no friendships because her life could not be disturbed by them. She lived a pretty lonely life. This is how sleep rituals can interfere with life and can be a symptom of an imbalanced system trying, at all cost, to rebalance itself. But the ideal state that will get you to go to sleep every time is a myth. It doesn't exist. Instead, trying to attain it makes the other dynamics and systems in life feel too delicate and protected to truly engage in life.

I was curious about what was going on beneath the surface, because we can treat insomnia with all kinds of things, but until we located the root cause of Pere's imbalance, I knew nothing would stick. She had her work life, which sounded like a pretty routine—if stressful—job as an assistant to a floor manager. It wasn't until we entered the second part of the hour that she talked about trauma from her past job: She had an affair with her supervisor, was fired, and, when she fessed up to her husband, he divorced her. She was far from over the frustrations she felt about her destiny.

The next time she visited, the conversation went deeper into her past. As is typical of anxiety-laden patients, she had spent most of nighttime rehearsing what she wanted to tell me.

Being raised the only child of ambitious parents, she was told what to do and when to do it throughout her young life. Her days were kept to a routine of house maintenance and school. She revealed a fearful time trying to satisfy her mother about her grades, which as I expected, she had made all A's except for math. Although she graduated from college with a major in history, she never applied for a job requiring higher than a high school education, probably because of her fear of failure. She had married as soon as she got out of college, to a school friend who was selected by her parents as her best choice, so she went along with the family plan.

When I was finally able to question her about the affair and her divorce, she described being a victim caught in a typical power issue in which her boss made it clear that her performance appraisal would depend on her willingness to share her body. She relented to his wishes, the relationship was exposed by a coworker, and she was fired. She confessed to her husband and he kicked her out of the house, filed for divorce the next day, and has never spoken to her again.

Pere had tried psychotherapy three times before, never with much success. She complained about her therapists (which I felt would sooner or later be my fate) because they wanted to focus on her relationship with her mother, who had passed away the year before. But she tired of reporting her simpering disgust, which never resolved her "real problem" of sleep, or rather, lack thereof. It was clear that talk therapy wouldn't get us far.

THE PLAN TO REBALANCE YOUR SLEEP RHYTHMS

Like Pere, when you're not sleeping, your brain and body decays due to lack of restoration. Your whole system becomes toxic, which is a problem in itself. Additionally, you don't have very much mental energy for true insight into your issues so you can sleep naturally. You can go to a therapist and talk twenty-four hours a day for a year, and not get anywhere, because there's just not enough energy in your system to change. True insight doesn't come from intellectual capacity alone, it comes from a mentality that can see the connections between the all the dots of your various traumas, stressors, and issues that are participating in imbalance.

This why the first thing we need to do to help you sleep is build back your energetic strength and balance the rhythms in your system. Otherwise, you're going to be more frustrated than ever and the degeneration will continue to affect your whole being—especially your immune system—as all efforts at remedies just spin out from nothing. When circadian rhythms are violated, it creates a mixture of conflicting currents of confusion within the mind. It's like being in an ocean where stormy crosscurrents are blinding in all directions, leaving you with no control over where you go. As a psychologist, I gave Pere a performance anxiety diagnosis, with underlying depression. However, her rhythms needed to be modified in order for her to have the energy and clarity for change. Only after the inner storm subsides can you see where you want to go, make changes, think through your problems with a fresh lens, and begin to organize your life in a more productive way.

The first phase of your rebalancing is to adjust your night-and-day orientation. There are three steps in this initial process: sleep hygiene, relaxing to sleep states, and entering the vulnerability of sleep so you can release control to a deeper consciousness. Like Pere did, you may resist these steps, but they are all necessary.

Setting the Time and Place for Sleep (Sleep Hygiene)

Make a commitment to set appropriate hours for sleep. You need to decide which part of the day you want to focus on restoring (sleeping), and which part of the day you want to be active. Your sleep period needs to be at least eight or nine hours long, consistently, if you are an adult. Teenagers and children need even longer periods. You can add some hours of relaxation or napping in addition, but you need to have at least eight to nine hours of consecutive sleep so your brain enters a Delta state. This is the time required to go through a complete restoration of your body and mind.

When this time arrives, go through a process of making your environment suitable for sleep, where you won't be disturbed. Here are some ways to do that.

- Have a comfortable bed that you only use for sleep or sex. Don't use it for anything else, especially not for discussions or arguments with your partner. When that happens, the bed becomes host to a significantly different experience than sleep.

- Set the temperature a little cooler than average, because your body needs to cool down during sleep.

- Turn off the television, cellphone, and the lights.

♦ Have some boundary for sound, like a closed door.
If you live in a loud city, play a white-noise machine
or an app with rhythms like ocean waves, wind, or
the gentle babble of a brook or stream.

This is not the time to go out and play, watch television,
or call a friend. It is time for you to focus on one thing—
resting and restoring. Pere did not want to set her hours of
sleep because doing so reminded of her mother's control, but
she agreed to try anyway. And in the process, I observed a hint
about what her deeper problem likely was.

Winding Down into Sleep with Relaxation

About an hour before bedtime, plan to engage some relaxation
strategies. You may be like Pere and resist, saying, *"I've got too
many worries I have to work through. I just can't go sleep because
I have to deal with tomorrow. I have to take the time tonight to
figure out what I'm going to do tomorrow."* That is disastrous. You
can't do that, because your brain is going to wake into its upper-
level consciousness in order to deal with the problems. Getting
back down to a lower level of sleep is then really difficult.

If you are too wound up to relax yourself, you may be
like Pere and need some brain training to enter relaxation
frequencies. The EmWave (available on www.heartmath.com)
is a biofeedback app in which you use breathing techniques to
evoke brain changes that you can monitor on your phone. The
goal is for the readings to show that your brain frequencies are
reduced down as close to Delta as possible. Most people can
do this with circle-breathing techniques, where you basically
breathe in and breathe out for the same count. As you exhale,

you also relax your muscles, such as your shoulders and legs. Breathing controls everything: your brain, body, and heart. So you just need to learn how to breathe in a specific pattern that lowers your frequency of consciousness on the biofeedback app readings.

An image can help you get into this lower level of consciousness, like being held by your mother or being sung to by your father, or calling up some other comforting memory. Over time and practice, the biofeedback system's reinforcement will train you to "shift and replace emotional stress with emotional balance and coherence," as the HeartMath website describes it. This is how Pere gained some control over her brain. Eventually, she could lay in her bed, do the exercise, and feel herself get closer to the Delta state. With training, she knew experientially that she was maintaining it and no longer needed the app to tell her.

You can also aid relaxation with music. I have produced a lot of music because we know through studies that listening to rhythms, such as lullabies, makes a big difference in our experience. A composition I produced, called "Relaxation with Flute" (available on www.mindbodybylawlis.com) uses a Native American Flute. I've found that wind instruments contribute a sense of breath and feeling light. Listen for at least a half-hour, and even the whole night through. Music is soothing to the mind and body. Its relaxation power is recorded in the bible: David played the lyre for King Saul so he wouldn't be tormented by thoughts and could sleep.

I was surprised when Pere reported that she would fall asleep after a few minutes, but she had the insight that as long as I was in charge and she wasn't responsible, she would resent the power of the music. We had work ahead, but in the meantime, she located a friend who would put a second music composition that I created on a loop for the night, called *Entropy*. This music evoked Delta frequencies all night, allowing her to follow her sleep stages according to the tides of the night.

If you live with someone, share a bed, or know anyone who is wonderfully generous, they can also help you relax before bedtime. Ask someone to read stories to you, just like your parents did when you were a child. Lay back and receive a massage, or at least a gentle rub. Feel specific muscles relax, one by one. If you live alone, you could listen to an audiobook as you lay under a fluffy, fuzzy, and otherwise tactile blanket.

Surrendering to Your Unconscious Mind

Through sleep, your unconscious can benefit your consciousness. Research shows that, if you're in a Delta sleep consciousness, your brain will "spindle up." Basically, little spindles come up that contain information. It's a long jump, but I think these are entry points into your consciousness, because my data shows a correlation to higher intelligence scores if dreams and other unconscious messages rise into awareness. I personally use nighttime dreams to solve math problems. This is also what I do when I write; I germinate the story I want to create and then I sleep on it. During the night, the details of the story come into view. When I wake up, I write down what I discovered. This process aided the discoveries and inventions of Thomas Edison and Einstein.

Sleep has at least five to seven different stages that you pass through while diving down into deep sleep and then coming back up. Throughout the night, you're going in and out of these stages. Usually around stages three to four, the focus is on your muscles as those are repaired. Then you go a little deeper to repair psychological issues. Then you might come up to a dream sleep in order to symbolize those issues and experience a way of processing them. You awake with a symbolic formula, and you may or may not know what it means. Just because you might not remember them doesn't mean you're not dreaming; sometimes the symbols are so obtuse that you can't bring them into waking memory. Some don't make any sense right away, though you may understand them as the day goes on. In the morning, it's good to talk about your dreams or to write them down.

If you're on sleeping medication or you're using alcohol or marijuana to sleep better, it will prevent you from going through the stages of regeneration. The substance might knock you out, but it keeps you at the top level of sleep and, as a result, you aren't experiencing the restoration you really need.

To access all levels of mind, you must open up to information from your unconscious—without defense. You need to be willing to be vulnerable and release control. When you go to sleep, you are allowing your brain to go into entropy, into chaos and disorder. Instead of focusing on survival, it allows other things to mix in—including divine messages. You must trust your sleep, because it will not only reveal things, but it will resolve things as well. That's its purpose, to resolve tension and toxicity in your life, whether emotional or physical. Let your sleep patterns resolve problems through unconscious processing.

With her performance anxiety about going to sleep, Pere just couldn't give up control, so it was hard to surrender to such chaos. Her ego battled to control all the thinking because, as I was finding out, she was afraid of allowing anything or anyone else gain an upper hand. She didn't want to enter vulnerability or weakness, which basically maintained self-esteem issues. But with her sleep hygiene and relaxation music, Pere began to sleep. This is what mattered. From there, insights could arise.

YOUR REAL STORY EMERGES

Soon after gaining a few successful nights of sleep, Pere's story about her relationship with her mother began to change. It turned out she was jealous of her mother and saw no value in her parenting. In her young life, Pere acted out with passive-aggressive behaviors. For example, frequently when her mother would ask her to perform a chore, such as washing dishes or taking out the trash, Pere would act incompetently on purpose—spilling dishwater all over the counter, breaking dishes by dropping them, or dragging the trash bag until it ripped open. The consequence is that she never completed a task and her father would step in to support her. This led to arguments between her parents, which pleased Pere. Along the way, she also revealed that she had seduced her boss, rather than the other way around. For that, she blamed her husband's lack of attention. The human resources department lawyers feared she might sue the company, so she got a year's salary to leave the company, hence she gained a long vacation as a reward she did not plan.

This kind of honesty led Pere to realize that she was not the innocent flower she pretended to be. Rather, she was actually a powerful woman who played her games with great skill. To her credit, she admitted that she did not receive the satisfaction she wanted.

In the same way, as your system rebalances, your thoughts and perceptions will become clearer. You will face deeper insights and messages into your self, your life, and your sources of imbalance. Seeing these things can be hard—you might see things you would rather not see and feel things you would rather not feel—so it helps to speak to a psychologist or friend who can encourage you.

If you want to return to getting full nights of restorative sleep, it does take some courage. For example, you might discover you don't actually like your mate as you realize just how much she reminds you of your mother. You might have disturbing dreams about killing your parents or shooting your husband. It might scare the heck out of you, but letting these things surface will ultimately help you understand the feelings you keep hidden—even from yourself. Essentially, once you gain more intellectual capacity by sleeping, you are going to discover things that you'd like to change. This might at first seem like a threat, but it is actually an opportunity that—as Pere found out—is a key to the healing journey.

FINDING RESOLUTION WITHIN

To help Pere enter her inner depths, I arranged for her to spend three hours in a sensory deprivation chamber, not expecting her to be able to stay that long. Pere stayed the entire three hours and requested even more time, but she needed to schedule another appointment. For the next month, she did this every week. Her eyes started to glisten and, although she did not seem pleased, she was obviously resolving something in the chamber.

In solitude, we all experience a kind of independence. Alone with your own attitude, thoughts, and values, you can begin to examine things within your own system and your own standards, instead of following the rules of any other person. You can become your own person. There is a lot of freedom in solitude, and it allows you to become more of the person you want to be. Within the human spirit, there seems to be a drive toward growth, toward being the person we want to be or were born to be. This happens without having to be reinforced or taught or therapized. In solitude, the universal rhythm of natural growth will resolve things.

Once in your sensory deprivation chamber, all you need to do is listen to yourself. Just let yourself hear your thoughts and feel your emotions, surrendering to the freedom of whatever arises. This freedom to explore is your birthright, and it will lead you back to who you are and evoke healing love from the divine.

After four sessions of this inner listening, with tears in her eyes, Pere whispered, "We forgave each other." When I asked her to explain, she said, "My mother forgave me for being a bad daughter, and I forgave her for being a bad mother." Then she was silent, got up and left the office, smiling, but with tears still flowing.

We had a couple more sessions where Pere discussed her insights, and she continued with the sensory deprivation experiences. She would call and report every once in a while, but not make an appointment. She had found her resolve by herself, and I remember one thing she said that clarified everything for me: "I am glad not to have to destroy my mother every night."

A year later, Pere stepped into my office, not to seek counsel, but just to report her pride that since our time together she had gained weight and taken a new job. She had found her "groove" and was enjoying attention from men. Once she gained insight into the core cause of her inability to sleep and resolved her fraught relationship with her mother in the sensory deprivation chamber, her rhythms found their own balance. She has been sleeping deeply ever since.

SLEEP IS ESSENTIAL TO YOUR PHYSICAL HEALTH

The circadian rhythm is one of the most important natural rhythms humankind has to align itself with because it influences our entire body-mind system. Like Pere, if our sleep is out of balance, we simply cannot muster the energy to change or adjust to the conditions of our lives. Our well-being is completely dependent on accomplishing good sleep health.

As one of the cornerstones of neurological treatment, balancing circadian rhythms helps the brain recycle toxins and waste accumulated through the demands on it. Just as our muscles have a system of cleansing themselves when they tire and build up lactic acid and dead cells with the *lymphatic system*, the brain has its own system, called the *glymphatic system*. Studies have shown that this system works best when we are asleep. If we are sleep deprived, the cleaning process breaks down and neurodegeneration occurs, which creates an environment that supports proteins like the beta-amyloids and tau associated with Alzheimer's and other dementia (Ehsan Shokri-Kojori, April, 2018).

My own research has shown that we are rarely taught how to sleep well. This is significant because we get one to two hours less sleep on the average than we did fifty years ago, with the invention of electric lights and our society's use of twenty-four-hour work cycles. Unless we can rebalance circadian rhythms, we are headed for major disaster, from the inside out.

THE ROLE OF SLEEP IN PSYCHOLOGICAL AND SPIRITUAL GROWTH

The unhealthy results of poor circadian rhythms are especially tied to brain disorders, which are obvious to anyone suffering from them. This makes it abundantly clear that, in addition to healing and preventing disease, sleep also supports psychological and spiritual growth.

Having been as a student of the intellectual giants of psychology, I have recognized that Carl Rogers was right when he postulated that humankind has an internal potential for growth and learning. As a result, his therapy model for counseling provides a safe place for patients to discover insights for themselves. They will find solutions through their own capacities. The counselor simply supplies empathy, caring, and genuineness to help patients recognize their strengths and choose the directions for their own self-investigation. The patient's own internal motivation toward health can provide the intellectual and emotional capacities needed to find the correct path to balance. In his conceptual framework, the energy the patient needs for this process of self-discovery arises from matching their real self to their Ideal Self. This is exactly the process that Pere went through. It is clear that as her circadian rhythms were reestablished, her brain lobes functioned better and her problem-solving abilities increased dramatically.

YOU CAN SHIFT INTO CIRCADIAN ALIGNMENT

By reading about Pere's struggle for joy and peace, your internal drive toward health can become apparent. All she needed was to be given some basic skills and a safe environment for her to progress in her journey toward health. In life, we all have adjustment periods that seem to be designed to make us miserable. There's never a time that you can coast in life. About the time we think we've got it made, something happens and we need to readjust all over again. You may be in an accident as an innocent bystander, and your whole life turns upside down. Relationships come and go, because they seem to have a purpose of their own. You may be facing a divorce from the most beautiful, wonderful person you know, simply because it's time to change. You need to make adjustments all along the way. Some can be major, most will be minor.

If, instead, a fixation happens and you get stuck in one of these periods, you've hit what I call an *adjustment barrier*. For example, you may remember the good old days of being a football hero in high school and remain there. You wear the same clothes, talk about the same things, and your development as a human being stops because that's when you got your biggest hit of self-esteem. As a result, you will become imbalanced and experience things like insomnia because you're not making an essential shift. To heal, we need to adjust in a fluid way as the stages of life happen.

Once Pere started sleeping again, her adjustment barriers were relieved and she could go further into exploring her mental, physical, and spiritual patterns. As her body regained the ability to restore itself, she could manage stress again—which built up the courage she needed to deal with her inner demons.

There is no doubt: Like Pere, you will run into another challenge in life that will cause imbalance in your body and brain, simply because that is how the experience of the human spirit was designed. Things change, our bodies age, weaken, and transition to another existence, based on our culture and expectations. Our ability to balance our system along the way is based on many things, but by attuning ourselves to the rhythms of our earth home and our inner wisdom, we can discover a guide for maximum performance and happiness.

CHAPTER 5

PAIN RHYTHMS AND OPIOIDS

There are no gains without pains.
–Benjamin Franklin

Our human body-mind system has always needed to manage physical pain. That may seem obvious when you imagine our ancestors hunting gigantic beasts and incurring injuries, or when you consider all the aches—minor and major—that you've endured in the course of your life. But it seems that, today, we have completely forgotten that our systems have a natural, built-in pain-management process. Instead, we have become dependent on medications like opioids to feel relief— which is a sad reality because in the long term, opioids actually inhibit our body's natural sources of relief. All we need to return to the healing rhythms of our own processes are a few skills, which are simple and ancient, but we have left them behind in the medicalization of health.

The rhythms to deal with pain are so ingrained into our bodies that they happen almost completely unconsciously. When we experience tissue damage, messages are sent to the spinal cord, where nerves stimulate the brain and the cortical central nervous network. The brain decides how to act in order to avoid further tissue damage, and we have little conscious control over its decision (think of the reflex that pulls your hand away when you touch a hot stove). Next, endorphins are released, which are neurotransmitters that move between the neuro-connections throughout the body. These substances block the transmission of pain messages to our awareness, at the brain level. Endorphins are our natural painkillers. You can witness them in action if you just pinch your skin hard enough for it to feel painful. Allow sixty seconds to pass. Your endorphins will activate and you should feel a reduction of the pain sensation, even though you are still pinching yourself.

If you were to take an opioid medication to ease the same pain messages, a cascade of negative adjustments occur as the brain attempts to deal with pain in relationship to the presence of the opioid. You see, opioids are parts of our receptor systems innately, ready to receive neurotransmitters such as endorphins. However, when additional stimulating medications are inserted into our neurological system, the receptor sites expand to accommodate the increased flow. With the expansion of receptor sites, we require more and more stimulating substances and end up needing more medication that we respond to less and less. This leads to a vicious cycle of opioid dependency. As a result, we experience more pain and accompanying anxiety because we have disrupted one of our body's most basic rhythms.

LIFE HABITS THAT LEAD TO PAIN

No one knows the downward spiral of opioid dependency better than Roy. In a true American success story, Roy had worked himself up from a foreman position overseeing the assembly line of automobiles to a corporate executive level, complete with a corner office where he sat at his desk all day. The steady streak of promotions was justified by his production successes, and he was proud of the support and pride his company showed for his work.

Soon, he began to understand the costs of the sedentary nature of his position. While he was on the assembly line, he had been active. Consequently, he was better conditioned to deal with pain because his body was more physical and better balanced. When he began sitting at his desk all day, and favoring his right side, his musculature got out of balance.

After a year or so in his new role, Roy began to have back pain. Sometimes it was so severe that he had to use a cane just to make the walk to his desk. He began to lose sleep, worrying about whether to consider medical leave, so he finally went to the doctor for an evaluation. The doctor told him that it was likely a muscle spasm and referred him to physical therapy. With this assurance, Roy did his physical therapy exercises as often as he could, but saw no significant improvement. Weeks turned into months, and Roy felt less and less energy—to the point that his performance on the job was suffering. At another visit to the doctor, he was referred to a neurosurgeon for a thorough evaluation. The result was a discovery of a significant bulge in his lumbar spine. Surgery was recommended.

Thing is, we all have bulges in our spine—every one of us—by Roy's age. That's not something to operate on. Generally, a rule in orthopedic surgery is that you don't operate on pain, because it is always mysterious, you operate on function. Ray got on the slippery slope of our medical system and into the hands of a naïve surgeon. Before he knew it, he was having a surgery that wouldn't ultimately solve his pain problem…and that introduced more factors that cause pain, like scar tissue and missed work.

The surgery was deemed a success, with a disk removal from the spine where the nerves were irritated. Roy was sent for outpatient physical therapy for six weeks. He felt relief and optimism…only to find that the pain returned worse than before. Another evaluation revealed a collapse of the same disk problem, plus protrusions of upper disks, so a multiple-disk fusion was recommended this time. Again, the doctors claimed surgical success as his back healed and the fusions of bone occurred as expected. But the recovery time used up all of his sick leave at work. To add to his worries, he was replaced in his position, but promised a job would be awaiting him as soon as he was able to work again.

Rehabilitation was harder for him this time, as he attempted to strengthen himself while enduring the pain of the surgery procedures. Throughout the process, doctors prescribed opioid pain medications. With a constant dosage, Roy felt strong enough to appear for a work evaluation and qualified for "sedentary" status. The job that was available for him was a file clerk position at a lesser salary. All in all, Roy was lucky—he still had a job and an employer on his side. Most people who fall into the downward spiral of opioids cannot work.

THE TRUE COST OF THE OPIOID DEPENDENCY EPIDEMIC

The opioid epidemic is infiltrating work offices across the country. A study released in March by the National Safety Council reveals that production and other work-related parameters have been negatively impacted by opioid dependency in more than 70 percent of workplaces. The data is consistent that the drugs are initially used for pain and prescribed by a physician. This number, although staggering, is considered conservative because most companies do not test for prescription drugs.

More than a million working adults are currently missing from the U.S. workforce, and experts are blaming the opioid crisis. Princeton University's economist Alan Krueger released a study in August 2017, attributing a 20 percent drop in the labor force participation rate for prime-age men between 1999 and 2015 due to the opioid epidemic. This means there are roughly 1.5 million working-age adults who are currently not working. NPR reports that there is a direct link between this statistic and the epidemic of drug use, specifically for the management of disease groups. Forty-seven percent of this group started using these drugs for pain management (Norsworthy, 2018).

On a more individual basis, every day, more than ninety Americans die after overdosing on opioids, costing important lives, as well as placing an economic burden on society. The Centers for Disease Control and Prevention estimates that the cost of the abuse of these drugs alone is $78.5 billion per year, only to possibly increase with the availability of non-prescription, addictive pain relievers across the nation. *Eight to twelve percent of patients develop pathological dependency.* A STAT analysis predicts that the annual death toll from opioid dependency will rise more than 33 percent between 2015 and 2027, which implies that more than five hundred thousand people could die from opioid abuse over the next decade. Do note that deaths from medical prescriptions alone greatly outnumbered deaths from heroine from 1999 to 2016 (Sanders, 2018).

The history of this situation can be traced to the 1990s when the pharmaceutical companies convinced the medical community that "patients suffering from real pain would not get addicted or dependent on opioids." But the reality is vastly different from this promise.

- Roughly 21 to 29 percent of patients with opioid prescriptions misuse them.

- Eight to twelve percent of patients develop pathological dependency.

- An average of 5 percent of the patients transition to heroin.

- In 2015, about two million people in the United States suffered from substance abuse disorders related to opioid dependency, and over a half-million suffered from related heroine abuse.

The biological risk for getting yourself into danger is very real, and quite high. The human body already has a massive array of internal opioids that a number of bodily functions depend on for management, such as pain and stabilization.

These proteins are considered to serve as the earliest evolution in the brain. Consequently, there are masses of opioid receptors on the brain stem, *pons* and *medulla,* which control the rate of breathing correlated to levels of O2 (oxygen) and CO2 (carbon dioxide) balances. Sensing the increases in CO2, the *carotid body* (neck cell cluster) might depress our breathing patterns to be deeper, or increase them to be more rapid, to respond.

A dose of opioid medication can suppress the throat's gag reflex, which in turn, can cause a drop in blood pressure or trigger a shift in heartrate variability. Moreover, these drugs can further dilate blood vessels and cause digestion issues, resulting in constipation and possible gut dysfunction.

An opioid overdose happens when there is a buildup of CO2, which causes *pulmonary edema*, an excess of fluid in the lungs. This condition can stress the system if it cannot generate enough O2 to clear this congestion, and the body quickly spirals into trouble. For example, a fast-acting opioid, fentanyl, can cause paralysis in the chest and, within seconds, death can occur. (Science News, March 31, 2018). These are the risks, and my hope is that by understanding them, you may decide to step out of this vicious cycle.

OPIOIDS ARE A TICKET TO HITTING ROCK BOTTOM

It's a sad reality that we often need to hit bottom to realize the extent of our problem—and opioids easily take people there. After Roy's return to work, his life devolved into a kind of hell. The file-clerk role was a demotion for Roy and was actually harder on him than the executive role because he had no assistance, which meant less time to pause and stretch, and required more walking time. His pain medication would work up to four hours and then his pain would grow worse. He kept his opioids close to him all the time so he could maintain his dose schedule.

Then the worst news of all came: Due to new regulations on opioid prescriptions, his doctor withdrew his pain medications and left Roy on his own to deal with the pain. Roy panicked. He knew he could not handle his job without his pills, and he could never face his family if he lost his job. So he went to the street for a source. The street drug he could afford—since it was the cheapest—was heroin. His dependency quickly grew into a full-blown addiction. With that turn, his work performance deteriorated, along with his marriage. As his bitterness about the turns in his life grew, his addiction began to consume his attention. When he wasn't high, he felt suicidal.

By some mysterious act of grace, perhaps agreeing with research that it is more economically beneficial to bring good employees back to health than to lose them, Roy's company went beyond their responsibility and offered to pay for rehabilitation services. That's when he showed up in my offices to try the Psycho-Neuro-Plasticity (PNP) approach for opioid recovery.

WHY WE ARE AT A LOSS ABOUT OPIOID RECOVERY

There were no promises that Roy would turn around his life, largely because there are so few practitioners who understand this epidemic fully and know how to correct it. Some of the confusion is led by the fact that doctors tend to think of recovery from opioids in terms of alcohol addiction. This does not tend to work, as the alcohol recovery field has a tremendous variability of approaches and there are many unregulated programs based on unscientific data, poorly trained staff, and questionable ethical practices. But the problem also exists because alcohol addiction is an old issue and opioid dependency is newer, only becoming a serious issue since 1990. So there are many incorrect assumptions about the impact on our brains, bodies, and lives—and this increases the dangers of dependency.

If we map the spectrum of drug abuse, in general, as brain models on a linear perspective, substances used for pain and anxiety relief would be at one end and substances used for pleasure at the other end. Addiction can be defined neurologically as a pleasure-center satisfaction and can hijack the brain through pleasure-seeking substances. Most addictions begin in early life as a pleasure enhancer, stress manager, social interaction "lubricant," and self-medication for deeper mood disorders.

But opioid dependency requires a different brain model because it falls on the pain and anxiety end of the spectrum. The main reason for their use is relief and maintaining functionality. In order to maintain those functions, dependency can happen. Opioid dependency often starts in later adulthood, at the doctor's office, as a way to manage the symptoms of disease. Significantly, many of these disease problems result from lifestyle conditions, such as Roy's poor posture, poor muscle tone, poor diet, and stress. More truth is that, often, the disease, such as skeletal problems, and surgical procedures to deal with the problems, are usually healed fairly quickly. The pain problems happen in recovery. Scar tissue around the surgery site can be a big factor in the reduction or magnification of symptoms. Stress and overreactions, as well as having poor skills in pain management, can easily be traced to patient complaints.

THE RETURN TO YOUR BODY'S OWN PAIN-MANAGEMENT SYSTEM

Here are the steps that worked for Roy, and many like him, which can also help you to return to your body's own pain-management rhythms.

Get Off the Meds and Detox

The first thing to do is stop taking all opioids and get them out of your system. When you know that help is on the way, in the form of new skills and techniques you can learn to manage your own pain, detox from opioids—and even heroin—is not that bad. What makes it terrible is when there is no hope that the pain will get better. You won't feel good while you detox, but you'll only feel bad for about three to seven days.

It takes about seven days for the receptor sites to recede after the medications are taken away, most often increasing anxiety, and requiring the alternative pain management techniques I'll soon share. But if allowed to follow the innate recovery process, the opioid receptors will recede and the natural pain mechanisms—endorphins—can be naturally restored. This is why your perceptions of pain will recede after this point.

Your brain simply needs time to regain balance from the inflammations and cognitive issues related to the chemicals that were in your system, and ruling your life, for a while. Addiction causes severe imbalances in the brain: It overstimulates your pleasure centers and basically controls your rational functions, as all your attention is devoted to seizing sources for the drug. As a result, you eat badly and don't take care to sleep or hydrate, which can cause brain damage. To aid cell repair, you need a period of detoxification. I've found that for about 25 percent of patients, detox is all they need to feel an immediate relief of pain. Once off the opioid dependency spiral, their body rhythms recover their functioning and return to doing their job. I hope this happens for you.

Eat to Support Your Brain and Reduce Inflammation

As soon as you return to a beneficial level of judgment about how to care for yourself, I recommend following a diet for pain. It basically consists of high amounts of protein and complex carbohydrates. In Chapter 9, I'll teach you a lot more about the powerful effects of nutrition on your healing rhythms.

Learn Skills to Support Your Body's Own Pain Management

In addition to going through a rehab program for substance dependency, it is crucial to learn how to deal with pain by using the natural rhythms of your brain and body. To enhance the productivity and actions of your endorphin system, one of the important facts to remember is that endorphins are most active in the parasympathetic state—which is when we relax.

- Biofeedback can help you reach the stage of relaxation that has been shown to be most regenerative.

- Learning to relax fully will also help your sleep cycles. When you listen to certain music, the rhythms can bring sonic stimulation to help you enter the frequencies of Theta and Delta brain waves. This type of deep sleep is tremendously helpful to increase your endorphin production.

♦ Listening to musical rhythms can bring emotional balance as well as spiritual uplifting, which can support your recovery.

You can gain power over your pain. This may seem hard to believe, but you do have the resources within you to control it. So far, members of the medical profession have not taught you how to do it; they have just given you pills. So it's entirely understandable that those seem like your only tools. The truth is that your mind is a powerful tool that can control pain through imagery. Try this exercise.

INSTRUCTIONS FOR USING IMAGERY

Close your eyes and imagine the pain in your body as some kind of object. It might be a hot ball, a steel rod, a pitchfork stuck in the middle of your back, or a burning coal.

Visualize the object clearly. Focus around the periphery of the object, right on the edge of your pain. For example, if you see your pain as a pitchfork, put your attention on the edge of the metal. Then make that space around the object a little bit bigger, which you can use your breath to do. Exhale air and visualize it surrounding the object, filling the space around the pain. You are seeing more open space around the pain, and as it gets bigger, you will relax and your pain will start to ease.

Often, colors are involved in the imagery. A lot of people see their pain as being red, as in red-hot burning pain. Sometimes people see blue, metallic, or sharp colors like gray steel. With your eyes closed, look at the color of your pain as you breathe space around it. Watch to see if the color starts to change, perhaps from red to yellow, or blue to green. It doesn't matter what color you see, you just want it to change.

After this brief visualization, perhaps lasting a couple minutes, open your eyes and rate your pain level on a scale of one to ten. As they say, seeing is believing.

Using imagery to relate to your pain and to control it has documented physiological effects (Victoria Menzies, 2006). You will feel a difference in your body as the pain shifts in sensation and intensity. Essentially, you are experimenting with what it feels like to constrict, or contract, around the sensations of pain and what it feels like to expand around them to relax. These constriction and expansion patterns we have in our bodies each affect your autonomic nervous system differently.

You can witness vividly how things that make you wound-up about pain (like anxiety, anger, worry, rumination, and obsessive thoughts) cause you to constrict into sympathetic responses that cause more pain. And you can play with using your imagination to visualize the expansion of space around your pain, which will be soothing, cause you to settle down and even find peace. By doing this, you—yes, you!—are engaging your parasympathetic response to ease pain and enter the healing zone. You can use this imagery to completely transform how you treat pain because your most powerful ally in healing becomes yourself.

Retrain Your Brain's Pleasure Seeking

Once off opioid medication, your brain will still go in search of transmitters to send to the pleasure centers to combat irritation and associated displeasure. In your brain, the *nucleus accumbens* is the pleasure center that gives you happiness through a variety of sources, including food. I've found that people who tend toward addiction often, in a normal state, produce lower levels of important neurotransmitters in this part of the brain. It's important to acknowledge this in yourself, if it's true. Do you tend to be unhappy more than you're happy? If so, it's likely that when you find something that makes you happier, like alcohol or a drug, you may say, *"For the first time in my life, I feel normal."* Nobody likes to feel bad. So once you discover a substance that elevates your nucleus accumbens, you are more likely to become addicted to it to feel better.

Breathing But what happens is that, because the nucleus accumbens is part of the limbic system, it takes over your emotions and eventually takes over the frontal lobe—which is your executive functioning. Essentially, the substance hijacks the brain. Your conscience is affected, and you lose your sense of values as you focus on getting more of the stuff that makes you happy. The heart of the conundrum is that you make this cognitive mistake: *"If I don't use this substance that makes me happy, I'm going to be unhappy the rest of my life."* This line of thinking is a huge barrier to your recovery.

The good news is that this can be countered. The emotional dimensions in the limbic system can be altered or reset. Craving impulses and pleasure-seeking nerve constellations can be repatterned. Here are some methods that you can research to retrain your brain to become happier without taking opioids.

- Breathing exercises

- Sonic frequency biofeedback, like the BAUD

◆   Meditation

◆   Learning new things, like how to play a musical instrument

◆   Cognitive Behavioral Therapy (CBT)

Cut the Obsessive Thinking Loops

One of the critical areas of the brain in the process of opioid addiction is called the *cingulate gyrus,* which serves like a switchboard to call into action parts of the body to adjust to problems, such as irritations. It lies just below the surface of the outer cortex and connects to everything directly or indirectly, and its important function is to integrate sources. We are often aware of this activity when we are creatively solving problems cognitively because of the way it sources ideas.

When exposed to opioids, which are hijacking the pleasure centers, the cingulate gyrus begins to get bogged down and becomes inefficient. No longer does it serve as a center for creative thinking, but tends to get stuck looping itself in thoughts, in an obsessive-compulsive way. If you are in pain, all you may be able to think about is pain and finding methods of dealing with it, such as drugs. There is no room in your thoughts for alternative approaches because your brain has no access to problem solving. You can rebalance this area of the brain through rhythmic reset methods, which I recommend researching.

◆   Sniffing powerful aromas, like eucalyptus and other strong essential oil scents, can cut obsessive thinking loops in the moment.

- Listening to music rhythms can help make new connections to stir creative thinking and problem solving.

- Using light to stimulate the brain can shift obsessive patterns long enough to reset the creative processes.

- Breathing in patterns, such as alternative nostril breathing, can be extremely helpful as well.

Overcome the Trauma and PTSD Associated with Pain

A significant brain element in this process is called the *amygdala,* which plays a role in the development of Post-traumatic stress disorder (PTSD). This area is known as "the recorder of traumatic events," especially negative emotions. Injury and the memory of pain (which has deep anxiety associated with it) can be accumulated so tightly that memories may arise within you so strongly that your immediate reality is overtaken by a trauma response. As a result, you may re-experience the trauma repeatedly. Chapter 7 is devoted to resolving trauma, so you may want to read it next.

Try to Identify the Imbalance That Is Pain's Root Cause

While the actual cause for your pain likely seems mysterious, especially after piling on medical treatments and surgeries, it's still a good idea to continue the search. For Roy, an electromyography (EMG) revealed unbalanced muscles on his lumbar back alignment, which meant that the muscles on his right side were significantly more spastic and tense than the left side. This indicated an enhancement weakness of the entire left side of his body. His right side responded by compensating to support his structure. Since this issue was not the result of a stroke or neurologically caused, we concluded that it was habit driven. Roy was overusing the right side of his back to deal with his life needs and an imbalance occurred over time. In my work as a clinical professor for an orthopedic surgery department, I have seen this muscle imbalance and loss of muscle rhythm result in severe back pain. Whether this imbalance was the cause of Roy's initial back problems could be argued, but it was a part of the rhythm rebalancing needed for an eventual return to his life mission.

This is why it is important to not only repattern the brain, but also to repattern skeletal, muscular, and connective tissues that sense pain and irritation. These components also include blood flow, since *arterial ischemic* pain can be intense and oftentimes a source of migraine headaches and spinal pain.

Like a car when the brakes are used too often or inefficiently, they break down. If the body's parts are not used properly, they wear down. But unlike the car, the body can mend itself. As we get older, many of our body parts weaken, such as muscles and immune function. Too much of a certain type of food and we may become sensitive or allergic to it; therefore, our diets have to change. Too much exercise can cause inflammation and the need arises to change routines. Roy began doing movements that increased his flexibility and range of motion, and that corrected his spinal overcompensation to bring balance back.

DISCOVER A HIGHER SENSE OF PURPOSE AND RESPONSIBILITY

In any life challenge, we can nurture seeds of self-discovery and transformation. We call this aspect of healing "transpersonal" because it consists of the experiences through which we can find new paths for defining our lives. *Transpersonal* means "elements beyond the self"—those spiritual and non-materialistic realities that are personal to our existence, and can be understood better when symbolized in some form. This can be of a religious nature or culturally defined by our traditions.

So often, when people reach the state that Roy was in— living with pain they can't escape—they feel God is punishing them. The Latin root of the word *pain* means "penalty." In Middle English (spoken from the 12th to 16th centuries) the word indicated "suffering inflicted as punishment for an offense." This notion lives deeply within us.

While Roy didn't exactly explain it that way, he sure felt he was the victim of fate. Women tend to think more along the lines of, *"God doesn't love me anymore."* A lot of people who are in automobile accidents rail against God or their sense of a higher power, because one of the hardest things to accept in life is that something can be done randomly. We ask, *"How could this happen?"* Someone could say, *"Well, you just shouldn't have been there at the wrong time,"* but, on a deep level, we can't accept that. We seem to need for there to be a reason for something bad to happen. This can lead to a spiritual crisis that feeds our inability to recover.

I have back problems. The cause of my back problems is not heroic at all. That's so disappointing to me because I'm partially crippled and can't walk very well. It's not that I got injured saving a child's life or picking something up in order to help another person, or something like that—which disappoints me. I feel devastated that the cause was stupid, and yet it still affected me for the rest of my life. Like you do perhaps, I ask myself, *"Why me?"*

There is a follow-up question I always ask next. *"Why not me?"* Try contemplating that, and it can be part of your healing process. The injury might have happened randomly, but at the same time, it might be an opportunity to show who you are, to demonstrate the positive stuff you are made of.

Roy had developed the skills he needed to break free from his opioid dependency, and while he was proud of his accomplishment, as he well should have been, his true turning point came when he expressed to me that he no longer felt so alone. Yes, his family's support was coming abundantly, but so was his sense of spiritual support. During the difficult time when he had been weaning off painkillers, he began feeling surrounded by a gathering of spiritual entities. They did not communicate with him directly—the power of their presences alone made him feel like they were his team, who rejoiced in each step of success. He felt messages of love being passed to him.

There are many ways to access the presence, and assistance, of powers greater than yourself, and they all involve looking within. Meditation and prayer can help you rediscover yourself, and your passions, to help you find new goals in your life. Participating in meaningful rituals, like a vision quest, can give you new perspective on this chapter in your life so you can emerge with a clarified direction in life. Hopefully, this will inspire you to meet the next life challenge with a fortified inner strength.

EMBRACING RENEWAL ON THE OTHER SIDE OF PAIN

With all these resources, Roy grew more and more motivated to work toward meeting his short-term goals, like walking to meals rather than having them brought to him, and long-term goals, like going back to work. You will need to rebalance your body, to walk anew, to nourish your body differently, to dissolve isolation, and learn to adjust to your strengths instead of your fears. Achieving these feats is rewarding and pleasurable—Roy strived for them with enthusiasm, and you can too. These new routines have been shown to enhance cognitive abilities, decrease depression and anxiety, and to enhance supportive attitudes toward one another. Learning new things, such as strengthening and stretching techniques with musical stimulation, has enormous value, as intellectual stimulation can be transformative. Being a beginner can help us regain our sense of humor, which is when we begin to taste the power of a renewal experience.

For Roy, each step moved toward regaining healthy life rhythms, and his sleeping evened out so that once again he could get a full night's rest—which was essential for his endorphins to take care of his pain so he could return to work. The inner work that Roy did brought a sense of the renewal that comes with rebalancing and realigning with life goals. His personal self-esteem grew, and with some marriage counseling, his family came back to their own balance and sense of safety again. His employer rehired him back in a job that was customized for him, in the human resources division where he would work more with people than papers. He developed a company-wide wellness program, based on his own experience. In this way, he paid for his company's belief and confidence in him by improving its production through the resilience of its employees. Roy's work had a greater sense of meaning than ever before. His loss of balance, in which he almost lost himself, helped Roy explore the possibilities in life anew as he recovered. This renewal is at the heart of the healing rhythms of life.

CHAPTER 6

THE SADNESS OF LOW RHYTHMS

*If we open a quarrel between past and present, we shall find
that we have lost the future.*
–Winston Churchill

If you are feeling sad or low, it might bring relief to learn that
sadness—and even depression—are natural rhythms of life. Just
as there are peak experiences in life, in which we feel abundant
joy or elation, there are valleys when we come down deep into
our innermost selves. As you will see in this chapter, I have
come to embrace sadness for the gifts it offers us all.

While our culture would very much prefer us to remain
upbeat, positive, active, and extroverted all the time, your life
will be richer if you can learn to also embrace darkness, stillness, and introspection. My hope is that as you read you come
to realize that sadness can be a great motivator to change your
life. It can be a source of inspiration or a dive into the depths of
a mystery that has no answer. It helps us understand each other
and learn empathy as a way of bonding with others, since we
all need support in dark times. It doesn't feel good, especially

for our egos, and we often fear it, but I feel sadness happens for good reason.

Essentially, the rhythms of sadness can help you move beyond your current identity construct—who you have been so far—into a deeper sense of yourself and your place in the world around you. This needs to happen at least five times in our lives, perhaps more, as we mature through the stages of life. Sadness, and sometimes depression, happen when:

- We face the rules of society in order to learn, challenge, accept, or modify them.

- We struggle with who we are, often because we simply don't know what to identify with or as.

- We come to grips with our own shortcomings in order to live with another person.

- We have to take care of another person through their illness or challenge.

- We see ourselves weaken with age and face death.

All of these stages are normal valleys in life, which cause us to reflect and, therefore, can be the basis for creating new directions for our journeys. There are indeed some depressions that have a more pathological basis that blocks dreams and hopes, yet the ways through them are much the same. In both types, the EEG brain map depicts sadness as an imbalance of the two halves of the cortex. I like to extend this description out psychologically to mean that sadness results when the rhythms of our soul have become imbalanced because we are not aligned with our deepest truth. The discomfort of sadness and depression can be alarm bells that your pleasures are based on things of fake value, important to others but not to you, or sources of instant gratification without inherent meaning or worth. Your low feelings are therefore guiding you deeper into yourself so you can eventually emerge closer to your truth. In this way, sadness and depression are essential life rhythms that accompany joy and happiness—all offering you the potential to heal and grow.

So you can see for yourself how this plays out, I want to share three stories of how people mined their depths through sadness to uncover things that ended up enriching their lives.

A CHILDHOOD SADNESS THAT LIVES ON

Jane likes to say she was born at the wrong time, with the wrong family. She was the third born of five children, having an older sister by three years, an older brother by two years, and two younger twin sisters by three years. After their first two children, her parents lost their zest for attending holidays and school functions, so Jane was usually left without her parents to celebrate milestones and achievements. In fact, they saw little benefit to even bothering to punish her, much less praise her.

The space that was left by their inattention was occupied by her older sister, Dolores, who relished in downgrading any self-esteem Jane might have found in the household. Jane lived a Cinderella story without the angelic figure to save her. She washed all the family's clothes and dutifully hung them out to dry on the clothesline—of course, she never did them correctly or as expected, especially the ironing. Jane's duties also included making breakfast for the group, who each had special needs and tastes, so she inevitably ended up disappointing someone. As a result of all the criticism, Jane came to feel she was a disappointment.

What bothered her most was not the demands that were placed on her time and energy, it was the lack of a role or identity within the family, other than being their servant. Her parents often discussed the fact that they birthed a perfect girl (Dolores), the perfect son, and the rare gift of twins. Jane was never on that roster of contributors to the family prestige list. In reality, Jane was more often described as the "problem" who had to be reminded of her status. They delighted in embarrassing her by pointing out she was wearing the wrong dress or hadn't brushed her hair. She heard whispers between her mother's friends when she was thirteen, saying they thought she would eventually get pregnant and have to leave the community for the sake of the family honor. This vision of her future as an outcast depressed her greatly.

When Jane did leave her family at sixteen, it wasn't because of pregnancy, it was an act of self-preservation. She left because she felt unwanted and decided that she could find a better life on her own—and she turned out to be right. She got on a bus late one night, arrived early the next morning in Dallas, Texas, walked to the state employment agency and interviewed for a job that afternoon. Maybe a guardian angel was on her side, because she landed a job as an assistant to an elderly lady who needed medical assistance, as well as clerical assistance for a book she was writing. Jane moved in with her new employer, so she did not have to find an apartment and could cook the strict diet her employer, Dr. Cobb, required. There was an immediate bond between the two and Dr. Cobb took an interest in her, since she had no children of her own. The job lasted for five years until Dr. Cobb passed. It had not been an easy job because Dr. Cobb was a taskmaster. She was controlling, changed her mind easily about what she wanted, and expected her assistant to jump at a second to meet her demands. Jane earned every penny she made.

Three things changed Jane's life as a direct consequence of this magical five-year period. Dr. Cobb had insisted that Jane complete her high school education and then encouraged her to make use of her new skills by applying at the local community college to become certified as a nurse. In her will, Dr. Cobb left her house and a significant amount of money to Jane. And more critical to the future, the relationship had given Jane a sense of self-confidence. Maybe Jane's early experiences of serving her family served some purpose, because Dr. Cobb was as demanding. But what was different was this: Dr. Cobb's expectation that Jane always do things well, even if she had never done it before, encouraged her until she gained a sense of self-respect and inner strength. As a result of these things, Jane could be considered wealthy, had a responsible job as supervisory nurse, and lived alone. She had no friends and everywhere she went, she went solo. Until she met Raymond and her life started another chapter.

Jane showed up for her first appointment with me thirty minutes early and waited patiently for her time, but never sat down. Rather, she walked in circles, silently mouthing some speech to herself. When I did see her, before I had a chance to ask what she came to see me for, she rambled through her life story. She apologized repeatedly for lack of proper etiquette for the situation. It turned out that she was suffering from bitterness about her early family experience and did not want it to spoil the promising relationship with Raymond.

A lot happens to us as we grow up. Sometimes we can feel stuck in our past, unable to move beyond anger and a sense of defeat. Freud called this "fixation," and when it occurs at an early stage of development, our emotional intelligence can get suspended in that immature state. *Emotional intelligence* is our ability to be aware of our emotions and the emotions of others, and to handle them well. Jane was fixated on her unloving childhood and on feeling unlovable, so she never matured her emotional intelligence. The past haunted her intently; even as she wanted desperately to enjoy her new relationship with Raymond, as his affection was abundant, she found herself unable to accept it. I also felt her past could certainly cloud her future, especially as she admitted being afraid of Raymond's intentions and worried she was being treated as a sexual object instead of a person with real worth.

Even when I offered her some methods to disrupt her thought patterns, Jane would repeat her anguish: "How can I let go of the fears and doubts? I don't feel anyone can truly care for or love me. I can't expect Raymond or anyone else to treat me like anything more than a basket case." Unless Jane could come to see herself as a person of real worth, there would be no resolution—which would be disastrous for their relationship.

DISRUPTING THE THOUGHTS THAT KEEP YOU DOWN

This tendency to get caught up in the same recurring, looping thoughts is also known as *rumination* and is a common way depressed brains keep us down. Sometimes, as for Jane, it shows up on brain scans similarly to the way obsessive-compulsive disorder shows up. If you are facing deep sadness, possibly from your childhood, you may be like Jane and not yet be ready to directly face the underlying fears and doubts. Here are some ways to disrupt rumination and looping thoughts.

Return to Balance Through Music

I recommended listening to the *Homeostasis* composition (www.mindbodybylawlis.com) to find a sense of balance and become familiar with it. Although Jane looked at me strangely, as if I was delusional for expecting some amazing changes overnight from listening to music, the effect on her was powerful. I received this note a few days later.

> When I started listening to your CD, I began to see vines on each side of me with beautiful white flowers, and the flowers were trimmed with lavender! The vines grew in front of me, moving and turning as they grew. All of these flowers on these beautiful vines surrounded me and continued to grow. The music continued to play. The flowered vines continued to grow and multiply. I was filled with joy and happiness for the first time in my life. My "inner home" filled out with rippling streams, birds, trees, moss, and a huge foundation. It was as if the music

was building this gorgeous place, but it was coming from inside of me.

Then there was a huge floral arch, and in front of the arch were two seats, for a king and a princess. The music moved me to a huge broken wooden cross with scattered rusty nails on the ground. The music then took me to see a place in the distance, a Southern-looking estate, and it began to burn. I sobbed intensely. The music brought me back to the garden and I was sitting next to Jesus and he said, smiling, "This is your home." He handed me the deed to my new home and I realized it was the first home that I had ever owned. It belonged to me. I felt happiness, joy, and completeness—complete with love and with peace.

I looked out to the distance, and the burning Southern-looking estate was just a smoking structure with only pieces of it still standing, and the sky above had a yellow-orange hue. I was back in my garden, my home, and Jesus and I continued to talk and share the music. There was no more hurt or anger or despair—just joy, happiness, and peace within me. I love my inner home. It's mine, it's beautiful, and I can go there whenever I want. My home is my soul, and it belongs to me and Jesus.

The music created a breakthrough for Jane that we could not manage in counseling sessions, but that is often how the healing process works. Certain music can offer a path to our unconscious through dreams and images that have symbolic significance, transpersonally or spiritually. These healing rhythms can bring insight and new visions for ourselves. Jane still listens to *Homeostasis* regularly. I invite you to integrate it into your life also.

Refresh Your Thoughts with Smell

Once Jane had a taste of happiness and balance, we worked on refreshing the feelings associated with her past. While the experience in the past was painful and negative, it's important to realize that the past doesn't need to rule your present with its misery. Smell is connected to an old, primitive aspect of our brain that is hardwired into parts that control emotion and memory. It therefore makes a great ally when it comes to disrupting thoughts of the past.

I asked Jane to close her eyes and think of her sister Dolores's voice or her mother's voice, as their abusive messages were running on perpetual repeat. When she had the imagery clear, I passed a tissue with a couple drops of her favorite scent of lavender under her nose and asked her to take some deep sniffs. Then I had Jane open her eyes and report what happened to the imagery. As expected, it had disappeared.

Aroma will reset your thoughts for about ten minutes, so you can use it whenever you want to escape the memories, voices, and messages from a painful past. The repetition will gradually retrain your brain's associative powers and you may well find that the past can soon arise in your mind without the misery it used to evoke. This is a powerful healing rhythm to break thought and emotional patterns that have held you back.

Defuse Emotional Memory with Biofeedback

I also used the BAUD with Jane. She called up a memory from her childhood and gradually turned the frequency knob on the BAUD until the intensity of the emotion increased significantly. With that frequency set, I instructed her to turn the disrupter knob until she felt the emotional memory fade away. You should have seen the smile on her face and how the light in her eyes shined as she felt freedom from her family's power. This was the last time they would haunt her.

EXPLORE THE ENERGY OF HAPPINESS

When we have grown up in the shadow of pain, we may not be familiar with how it feels to be happy. If your default mode is sadness and depression, you will return to it out of habit. Joyful feelings may be too foreign to integrate for long, so they remain extremely fleeting and unsustainable. You may even think happiness comes from the highest of highs—and chase those through extreme sports, dizzying love affairs, or even substances—never knowing that it can be experienced in simple moments of life. Once Jane had disrupted her painful thinking loops, and was curious about new possibilities to experience, I needed to teach her what happiness was. Again, I turned to sound.

Drumming for Inner Stimulation

With all my research into the power of drumming in healing, I tend to integrate drumming into a lot of protocols for various ailments. To help Jane deepen a positive connection with her inner world, I beat a drum at a frequency that stimulates imagery, which is about four beats per second. You can also beat the drum yourself and listen with eyes closed. Listen to both the sound and also what arises from within, especially the feelings in your body, any mental imagery, emotions, and messages. Jane's vivid imagery expanded her hopes into dreams for her life that she could look forward to pursuing. Previously, she had been too scared to have children for fear of repeating her family's abuse. But because she had seen how it's possible to shift those patterns from within, while listening to drumbeats, she connected with a desire to raise children with Raymond.

Establishing Your Rhythm of Joy

A variety of sounds work well for brain change, and another great one is the gong. It's sound is inherently uplifting, as it has been part of sacred ceremony since ancient times. I encouraged Jane to choose an instrument to play, and she chose my twenty-inch gonging symbol. At first, she soundly beat it with the same rhythm of four beats per minute, and then grew excited. With the goal of establishing joyful imagery, she defined her own rhythm, and smiled broadly as she discovered her own "joyful" setting. She played the gong for an hour, listening to both the sound and her experience within. Then she proudly said, "Now I know when my brain is happy."

Like Jane, you can explore sound and its healing effects on you. You don't need to be a musician and, in fact, the simpler the rhythm, the better it will reach your body and mind. In addition to a drum and gong, try a chime or a rattle. Whenever you want your brain to be happy regardless of circumstances, you can play with finding your brain's joyful frequency with sound. Over time and repetition, you will strengthen this part of your neurology and increase happiness within your whole being.

FEELING LOST, WITHOUT MEANING OR PURPOSE

All of us can feel adrift, directionless, and uncertain of our purpose. These periods in our life come and go with changes, losses, and failures—and they are marked by sadness and depression. They herald a time of introspection in which we ask ourselves big questions and emerge with reminders, or even new answers, for why we are living.

JJ's experience with loss of meaning is similar to other celebrities and people who experience great success. As a teenager, he had a couple major musical hits and some roles in movies, which brought him fame and money. JJ had no worries about his future; it seemed scripted for continual success. Each night was a party and all his bad behavior was excusable, even when he threw up on himself or passed out naked on the lawn. He had a million friends who glorified him and themselves with the freedom that his celebrity status provided. Girlfriends were plentiful and eager. JJ's story is common among young people who live off early success or their parents' money, and never develop a true sense of purpose or responsibility.

As JJ's twenties progressed, it all went away. The jobs dried up. Somebody else turned out to be sexier or more talented, and adulthood hit JJ hard. He may have grown a few years older, but in his brain, he was still sixteen years old. Out of touch with himself, and with no more songs to sing, he only had parties and drugs to uplift him. With the help of his talent manager, JJ made an appointment with me, but it had to be rescheduled until JJ was sober enough to be able to speak a complete sentence. Four broken appointments later, we had a face-to-face talk, and agreed on a mutual reality: JJ needed to sober up and detox until he actually wanted to change and grow up. He went to an inpatient rehab clinic for forty-five days.

A year later, JJ showed up at my office with sadness and depression written all over his face. He appeared more like a forty-five-year-old than a twenty-something. He spoke with an honesty I was glad to hear, felt an urgency to grow up, and wanted to figure out the life he was meant to live. I was convinced that his brain was stable enough not to waste our time, and his depression was a good sign that he deeply felt a motivation to find a place in our world in which he could develop true respect and honor for himself. The only way through this conundrum is to look within, and pray, for vision.

Shifts in the direction of our lives can come on slowly, as we realize we took a gradual turn that headed us off course. Perhaps you now see that you've been living out someone else's ambitions, or you put dreams aside to provide and care for your family. You may even see the sense in taking this detour, but your inner navigation system is now sounding an alarm through an empty sadness.

We can also be shaken awake by accidents, catastrophes, and great losses. Life suddenly feels like sand running through our fingertips and a deep part of us longs to make the most of it. The things that were so important recently—like the next promotion, the new BMW features, or who the murderer is on our favorite TV show—all fall away and we are left in a void that seems endless.

Like JJ, you can learn to listen to your soul's voice. You can pay attention to God or your higher power. This is not the time to avoid, pretend, or fixate on distractions; that will only deepen the looming feelings of oblivion. This is a time to be curious about yourself and courageous enough to explore how you can change for the better. We all have a challenge in life to find our niche and to become a member of a community, to find some joy in who we are—regardless of how much it pays or how much prestige comes with it. It's up to each of us to find this niche, or sense of purpose, for what we can do to contribute. It helps to arrange your environment in ways that support inner listening.

Remove All Stimulation

The deep immersion within your inner world becomes heightened in solitude and the absence of all distraction or stimulation—including everyday objects, light, and anything your senses might fixate on. Inner messages tend not to arise until we are in a state of receptivity. Because there was no sensory deprivation chamber near where JJ lived, he cleared out a closet, shut the door, and spent a night in it listening to my composition *Entropy*. The next day, he spent eight hours in the closet and on the third day, he was in it for six hours. It worked. In that time of listening to what is important to his soul, he rounded an essential corner.

He reported, "I'm closer to knowing what I want to be when I grow up. I want to help people, but I don't know how. Other than give money away, I don't know how."

JJ had more inner work to do, but he was set upon a mission to discover himself and his unique contribution to others and the world. You may experience deeper breakthroughs, through imagery, emotional release, or a spiritual presence, that guide you to answers about your purpose. If not, like JJ you may powerfully connect to the need to go on a quest for meaning.

Enter a Vision Quest: Wandering to Find Yourself

For JJ, this quest took the form of a trip. I encouraged him to wander for forty days, by himself, and because he was a celebrity, he went in disguise and with another name. He went to South America and wandered there, with the focus of exploring how he might help people in ways that went beyond giving them money. I eventually received a post card from him that said he had been reborn into a wonderful life, and that he had found happiness by giving to others what he lacked in himself.

Even if you cannot leave behind your responsibilities, job, or children to wander in another country, or even in nature, you can quest for meaning. Hold your intention as you explore new things with an open mind, pay attention to sacred "coincidences" that connect you with people and activities, and follow the inspirations of your heart. All this will shake up the routines that previously trapped you, introduce you to new ways of being and relating, and get you closer to changes that will make the visions that emerge manifest.

EVEN HABITUAL AND GENETIC DEPRESSIONS ARE WORKABLE

Some among us are genetically prone to unhappiness and others lack the ability to be sad or depressed. Personally, I would prefer to become depressed because it brings periods when I learn more about life. Yet many people, perhaps you, have a genetic predisposition toward depression, or have become deeply and habitually fixated on sadness. This is a very real and deep sadness that continues beyond a period of time and becomes the focus of all thought and activity or, likely, the lack of activity. This is when depression is clinically diagnosed. You will benefit from professional therapeutic help. Still, if you get so tired of feeling down that you decide to do something about it, there are healing rhythms that can reignite life's passions.

Nate was in such a state. He had been so depressed for so long that he had forgotten what it was like to experience joy. Even as a young person, he had no real memory of feeling happy or joyous. He mostly felt like an outsider in life, watching as people enjoyed holidays, games, and celebrations. He would participate, but never seemed to feel the way others did. In high school, it became apparent that he was stuck. His parents tried sending him away to camps and therapeutic boarding schools, and all it did was further isolate him.

When he came to me, Nate was twenty-eight and still living with his parents. As we spoke, I understood that he didn't like himself or his situation any more than his family did. He was lost and felt forgotten by God. What he needed was a primer in experiencing joy. He needed to learn what it feels like, in body, mind, and spirit, so he could build happiness into his neurology and choose activities that support it. Here are the ways Nate learned to be happy.

Check Your Genetic Code

I sent Nate for tests to see if he had a mutation in the methylenetetrahydrofolate reductase (MTHFR) gene. This is a gene which codes for an enzyme that breaks down the amino acids *homocysteine* and *folate*. When mutated, it can interfere with the enzyme's ability to function normally or completely inactivate it. The result can be mental health issues, including chronic depression. Because Nate did have the mutation, I recommended a nutritionist who worked with him on a diet and supplement regimen that could bolster his physical capacity for positive emotion. Getting tested can help you know if this is something that will support you too.

Stimulate the Experience of Joy with Music

I created a composition called *Neurological Stimulation for Joy*. We have found that, by listening to it and marching in place or around the room, such as a soldier would or someone in a marching band, you can enhance the body's neurochemical activity that results in feelings of joy. This is a great way to learn happiness and train it to be a neurological response to stimulus. Nate's first task was to march to this music two times a day, minimum.

Enhance Peaceful Feelings by Breathing

Nate was consumed by negative thinking, which led to mental and emotional paralysis. I taught him to find relief from tough emotions, in the very moments that they arose, by introducing him to the rhythmic power of his breath. Never underestimate the power of pausing to breathe. You can connect to the sense of peace that the breath brings by slowly and deeply breathing in for a count from 1 to 7 and exhaling for a count of 7 to 1. I recommend practicing this daily so you have a bodily memory you can call on in a tough moment.

Enhance Sleep Rhythms for Healing and Refreshment

Once you have practiced feeling joy and peace, a sense of inspiration and empowerment can begin to arise in your healing journey. Because Nate was feeling understood and had been introduced to his own capacity for happiness for the first time in his life, he became willing to try new things. You are likely to experience this also.

At this point, I recommend improving your sleep rhythms. Nate was playing video games all night long, which had disrupted his circadian rhythm. This further cemented the imbalances of his depression. I recommend that you read Chapter 4 in this book and give yourself the renewing gift of deep sleep.

Begin Exploring Life's Many Healing Offerings

Once you are feeling just a small amount better, start looking for activities that appeal to you. This book is filled with ideas for ways to engage healing rhythms in our bodies and world. Nate thought he might try yoga, and the real turning point for him came three weeks after he became a member at a local yoga studio. I prescribed that he take yoga classes five times per week for three weeks.

When he next walked in my office, Nate at first tried to hide a big grin. Then he came right up to me and hugged me tight. He said he had felt sore, tired, overwhelmed, angry, disgusted, and many other emotions in the past three weeks, but he kept his promise. He said he felt thankful that I took the time to understand him and ask him to find the inner strength to follow a new routine.

His next question revealed how far he had come from spinning his wheels all his life: "What's my purpose?" Nate is now a well-known yoga teacher with his own studio and students. He uses his studio to host sound-healing sessions where they play *Homeostasis*, *Neurological Stimulation for Joy*, and many more of my compositions. He has his own place, his own life, and though he isn't always happy, he does experience it from time to time—just like the rest of us. He has learned that it is okay to be sad, that there is nothing wrong with him. Now he is aware that happiness could be just a moment away. Maybe what's more profound than momentary joy is the enduring peace he feels after practicing and teaching yoga, in accord with his life's purpose.

HOPE FOR TOMORROW

Depression and sadness are a normal part of the human experience. It's getting stuck there that becomes problematic. There is a natural, seasonal rhythm of sadness that each of us experiences to inspire new understanding of ourselves and the compassion that can give others the support they need during these seasons as well. It's a terrible myth that if we are not happy, then something must be wrong with us. There is always hope for peace, love, and joy beyond the horizon of today, if we only bear our rhythms of sadness with dignity and understanding.

CHAPTER 7

RHYTHMS IN TRAUMA'S AFTERMATH

*Out of suffering has emerged the strongest souls; the most
massive characters are seared with scars*
–Kahlil Gibran

The natural rhythms of our lives take us through wonderful times, when everything flows well, and also painful times, when it seems nothing can go right. While you might prefer to subscribe to a more Pollyanna version of life, it can be healing in itself to accept that ups and downs, highs and lows, and peaceful times in between, will always be coming and going. Life is a bit dangerous, as there are indeed things in the universe that threaten us. Whether it's war, accidents, or people with harmful intentions, hard and bad things happen that traumatize us.

This chapter will show you how we're built to recover from trauma. As our ancestors faced adversity and survived, our DNA grew strong but not perfectly. We do get harmed and die from things unnecessarily when tools exist to prevent or treat them. Our personal mission is not to thwart disaster, as it is more likely to touch your life in some form than not.

Instead, we can focus on recovering in ways that strengthen us, so our children and our children's children have DNA with that same strength.

In a sense, we are all born traumatized. Being introduced to the world and breathing that first intake of cold air must be extremely painful for new lungs. We lose a loving womb in which every caring nurturance is automatically supplied, without our experiencing even a hint of need. To break that bliss is an unfair event and, as a result of being born, you entered a lifetime of earning your keep, getting through the misery of pain, and being a citizen.

Because trauma is experienced differently, depending on the person and their culture, expectations, past experiences with trauma, and goals for life, the path of moving through its effects rest largely with you. The stories I share in this chapter relate to battleground trauma and rape trauma, and my hope is that you will finish this chapter with hope and a sense of where to turn for the help that will most benefit you in your uniqueness. What happened, who you are, how you responded in the moment, and how you process it as time goes by determines how you will heal. Most likely it involves an event, or a series of events, that your mind cannot contemplate because of the horror or confusion you felt. Whether you were physically injured or not, the cognitive injury manifests as being unable to integrate what happened and adjust effectively.

What's more important than what happened, in terms of healing from it, is how you have responded. Trauma tends to shake up your whole concept of what the world is, what life is, and who you are. Things get turned upside down and you don't know left from right, up from down. Nothing makes the same kind of sense anymore. Instead of helpful thinking, you get stuck wondering things like: *How could this possibly happen to anybody, especially me? Did I cause it? Is it something I did? Did I piss off God? What did I do to deserve this?* When traumatized, we often modify our neurological integrity in ways that impair the normal, rhythmic organization of judgment and cognitive understanding of the world. Therefore, I find that recovery from a traumatic experience must include rebalancing brain patterns, in addition to encouraging psychological adjustment.

In this case, "talk therapy" or medication cannot be effective alone. Trauma affects our most primitive brain centers, and the evolution of language is new to our neurological development. Healing the cortex, or outer layer, of the brain with talk therapy will not work for trauma because there is a deeper source of imbalance. Even long after traumatic events, which are the imbalances of life affecting our innermost selves, the body and brain's rhythms can be restored to harmony.

RECOVERY FROM HORRIFIC EVENTS

Pete became a military man at an early age, largely because of the pride his family felt after his father achieved many honors during his career in the marines. He served for three tours and insisted on seeing action throughout to achieve promotions more quickly. He had a childhood friend, Tom, who followed him through training and tours with him. Being extremely close, they promised that they would take care of each other and that Pete would "never leave Tom behind."

On his third tour, although he had experienced the loud shocks of the big guns before, he and Tom were trained in a new weapon that sent bolts of earthquake-like waves through his body. He had major headaches for hours after they used the weapon. This would be the grounds for a promotion, so he did not complain about the side effects. He was excited about using this power against the enemy and immediately had the opportunity to demonstrate it.

Pete and Tom were sent on patrol to intercept possible enemy movement, but when they arrived, they were ambushed. Bomb blasts went off all around him, such that he did not know where to aim his weapon. At one point, he was ready to die and felt little fear. But then Tom tugged at his arm, saying something he could neither hear nor understand. He looked down at his friend and was shocked to see that his entire lower body was missing. Horrified by the sight, Pete's total mental and physical motivation immediately focused on saving his buddy's life.

Without any idea where the enemy was, nor any fear for himself, Pete pulled what was left of Tom's body on his back and started to run. His main thought was to run anywhere away from the thunderous sounds and pools of blood. When the medics found him, they described his behavior as raving and confused, and said that he was deaf. He kept asking for a doctor for his friend, who was already dead by the time they reached help. Pete was not injured, but was sent to the hospital for his mental state. Although he was informed that his friend had died, Pete would not acknowledge it and kept requesting help for Tom.

Pete was sent home with a post-traumatic stress disorder (PTSD) diagnosis. Even as he began to grasp the reality of what had happened to both himself and Tom, he did not cry and hardly showed any reaction when his family showed up at

Tom's funeral. He refused to leave marine life because he had no apparent injury and insisted on rejoining active duty, but this request was denied. While he did appear competent to perform the duties required of him, he was denied primarily because he was on psychiatric medication.

Pete spent most of his days being stoic and hiding his fears and self-doubts about being a failure. He was a stranger to his wife and tried to use whatever excuses he could make up not to attend family rituals, like birthdays and holidays. He overreacted to loud sounds and had constant nightmares. The night that he awoke suddenly from a dream and realized he was attacking his wife with a knife, mistaking her for the enemy, was when he decided to see if I could help. When he came to me, I insisted on seeing him twice a week because I feared that he might consider suicide along the path of recovery, but he didn't. As is universally true for healing, I found that I first needed to balance basic biological rhythms before we could turn to psychological and spiritual ones.

Recover Your Brain Function

If you are a soldier, or received an impact wound on your head during a traumatic event, your recovery may first need to address any damage done to your brain. Traumatic Brain Injury (TBI) can affect your feelings and behavior, which can persist despite your best efforts to heal. If you have a hard time controlling impulses, demonstrate poor judgment, experience a loss of social skills, changes in sexual behaviors, changes in self-esteem, impaired self-awareness, or depression, anxiety, or mood swings that just won't ease no matter what you do, you might want to visit a doctor for a brain scan.

Soldiers can develop brain injury from the intensities of loud sounds they are exposed to through explosives and cannons. I recommended that Pete experience some sessions of hyperbaric oxygen therapy (HBOT). A hyperbaric chamber is what deep-sea divers use to alleviate decompression sickness, which develops when they go deep underwater and come up too fast. The therapy consists of breathing pure oxygen in a pressurized room or tube, which reduces brain inflammation. This has also shown to significantly reduce PTSD symptoms. After twenty sessions, Pete's thinking cleared up and his depression eased.

Shift Brain Patterns Toward Healing

Pete's next step was an intervention with the BAUD in order to shift his brain patterns toward more constructive and optimistic goals. In a typical protocol, I used the pitch knobs to locate his emotionally obstructive imagery, which we found quickly, and then used the disrupt knob to decrease the neurological patterns causing him distress. He also found that frequency by turning the knobs himself. But the horrors and dangers of war he had lived through, as a soldier tasked with killing other soldiers, were not the thought patterns he was fixated on or found most stressing.

Instead, when Pete touched on the huge sense of responsibility he felt for Tom's death, he started crying and had trouble stopping, though he did manage to beg me not to write that he cried in a report. There was no need to speak much at all; I just listened to the pain over his loss express itself. We spent an hour and half just going from one emotional point to the next, as Pete grappled with his life, his God, his inner torture and, above all, his failure. By the end of the session, he was exhausted but felt relieved to express his grief and suffering, as long as I continued to reassure him that the emotional outburst would not be reported.

Weeks later, I felt Pete had made great strides toward healing his cognitive abilities and grief, so I offered to try the BAUD again. Though he felt some hesitation that it might trigger another crying session, he agreed. When we found the frequency of his emotionally intrusive imagery, he verbalized the confusion and fears about the battle and his loss of direction. He also described some of the emotional horror he felt the moment he saw his friend had only half his body and was dying. The frequency setting that disrupted these images brought a smile to his face. He immediately relaxed: his breathing deepened and his shoulders lowered, as if releasing a great burden. He just sat there and laughed for a while before he said, "I don't know what happened, but it went away. How could that happen? It just all went away."

Let Your Wisdom Emerge

Almost throughout Pete's treatment, he listened to the *Entropy* music composition to help him sleep. My hope was also that deep sleep would allow some wisdom to arise from his unconscious mind, as he had been experiencing nightmares. It's my belief that even nightmares are healing, as they allow us to access our raw fears and resolutions. As healing occurs, having access to our dreams brings bursts of insight that can give you a sense of spiritual guidance and destiny. This heightens your optimistic view that life can go on and bring good things once again.

One night, Pete had a dream of the great cosmic joke and woke up laughing. It was the kind of laughter when you just can't stop: tears come out your eyes and everything you encounter is also funny. When you look back on the joke, you don't know quite why you laughed so hard, but what's important is that a profound energy gets released that reconnects your being to healthy rhythms. Pete's laughter began in a dream when he was sitting with Jesus. Jesus cracked a dark joke about a soldier who got both arms shot off. This guy's main concern was, *"How the hell am I going to wipe myself?"*

What Pete got out of Jesus's punchline was the perception that we're on earth for only so long. The true joke is to think that we should get through life without struggle. Laughing at our human frailties, concerns, and even miseries showed Pete that he could take whatever comes in stride.

Laughter is best when it happens spontaneously and wholeheartedly, so there aren't any techniques that I can teach you. Laughter is physiologically important, as it changes your hormones and lowers your stress levels. Just be ready for anything that tickles your funny bone. There may be someone in your life who can make you laugh at anything, even the worst thing. Maybe there's a movie or comedian who gets you every time. Know the most potent, healing laughter comes when you can laugh about a really hard situation, like the one you're in. Doing that can change your perception of the world.

The rest of Pete's story is almost a magical. He explained his trials and struggles to his wife and eventually felt comfortable enough to discuss it with his children. He also talked to his father, who showed great empathy for his son's journey through hell. His confidence gained him a place back in active duty, where he reestablished a career path as a coach for younger solders. The last note I received from him said, *Thanks for resetting my sails.*

RECOVERY FROM BETRAYAL

Janis was a smart and pretty young woman who started life off with everything in her favor. She was raised as an only child with wealthy parents. The privilege of her upbringing may have led to an unawareness of the dangers of the world, which almost cost her life. At sixteen, she naturally became fascinated by boys and was the focus of their attention also. One such boy, Mike, was doing his best to add her to his list of conquests when he invited her to a hole-in-the-wall bar in a not-so-good part of downtown, where he and his buddies liked to hang out. She showed up, much to his surprise, because she was excited by him and curious to see another side of life.

As the night proceeded, more of Mike's friends joined the party. All were drinking and, when Janis submitted to taking sips of their beer and acted a bit tipsy, things got out of hand quickly. Noting that the guys were crowding around her too close, she started to leave, but they stopped her. She became afraid and thought about running, but her instinct lost the argument with the part of herself that wanted to be friends with Mike and insisted this was all part of being a cool girl. Not knowing what else to do, she relented to taking shots. When she was drunk, they led her to the back of the bar and into the stockroom. It was dark.

Suddenly, Mike became absorbed into another person without kind intentions. Janis found herself on a table, with her hands and feet held tightly. The men sang words she did not understand, but knew they were about her. She struggled mightily, but then became so frightened they would hurt her even more if she fought that her body went limp. This was when the mob tore her pants off and, one by one, raped her. They laughed and cheered each other on as they tore into her body. Mike was one of them.

The owner of the bar was in the front office when he heard yelling and arrived in the storeroom to find the aftermath of this horrific scene. The boys all ran out the backdoor before he could stop them. He immediately called the police, who took Janis to the station. There, she called her parents and, while she waited for them, she was given a rape-kit exam. A woman police counselor talked to her, consoling her and describing her rights.

When Janis's mother entered the room, her first words were, "What did you do to provoke those men, young lady? You are grounded until you are eighteen, as of right now!" She then turned right around and stormed out, leaving Janis in shock.

Her father meekly entered, gave Janis a slight hug, and guided her outside to their car. On the way out, he told the policeman at the desk, "We will not be pressing charges. It has been rough on us as it is. No need to drag this out in front of the neighbors and court." The next day, the car they had bought Janis was sold as punishment, and Janis was sent to her grandparents for the rest of high school, until she went to college in another state.

I met Janis in an addiction clinic after she had detoxed from heroin. She had been prostituting herself to fund her drug habit, and this was her fourth time through inpatient treatment. It did not require a psychologist to see she was very troubled. She freely shared that the rape at the bar was her reason for becoming a prostitute. In a twisted way of thinking, she had found some pride in a belief that she could make men do crazy things at her whim. However, she kept her mother's comment that night to herself...until Janis started changing her worldview.

Locate the Core Source of Trauma

Trauma can be complex and multilayered, so it's important to trust yourself to intuitively know what aspect of events wounded you to your core. This wound might be driving your behavior deep under the surface because it may primarily consist of the message you took away, rather than what horrible thing happened. You might fixate on this message, set out to avoid it by proving it wrong, or it may cause you to give up on life. When I asked Janis to share what was at the heart of her emotional trauma, she did not bring up the gang rape, but instead recalled her mother's hurtful accusation that what happened was Janis's fault. She blamed her mother for the trauma of being shamed, rejected, and—most of all—betrayed.

As Janis reached for more descriptive words, she explained that she could not wrap her mind around why, in that moment, her mother had announced to the world that Janis was a whore. She kept asking, "Why, why, why would she say that? I had no idea she felt that way about me, especially since I was a good kid, made good grades in school, and was even on track to graduate with honors. Why does she hate me that much?" Janis's world had become fixated on that one point, and her unresolved emotional hurt explained why heroine was her drug of choice. It took excruciating pain away for a while. Both the addiction and prostitution were the results of her shame and difficulty making sense of how her mother saw her.

After the detoxification cleared Janis's mind of heroine's influence, she had better insight into her demons. But years of numbing herself with it prevented her from expressing her feelings, so I had her build relaxation skills using the EmWave. As her firm guard against tough emotions relaxed, she started perceiving her situation better and could finally see how she was damaging herself. Her mother wasn't determining her choices. This broke the spell of punishing her mother by harming herself, and the door to healing opened.

Find Your Own Inner Resolution

When we become fixated on a harmful message, it becomes lodged in a primitive part of our brain called the *amygdala*. This part of the brain does not respond to rationality, so no amount of reasoning would help Janis stop reliving her shaming experience or acting against herself as a result of it. I encouraged a session with the BAUD in the hope of releasing Janis from her mental and behavioral trap. She found the triggering emotional imagery so quickly it seemed she was reliving that scene in every moment of every day. The disruptor frequency calmed her down immediately. She did not move as I encouraged her to breathe deeply. After several minutes, she lifted her head and smiled.

"She's gone," Janis said. "I am here and she is gone." Tears rolled down her face and she just breathed, as if to recapture the moment of her release into freedom. Then she turned to me with a childlike expression and said, "I still love her. I don't understand why she said what she did and sent me away, but I still love her." Sobs followed her words and I have to admit that tears came to my eyes also.

An essential part of treatment is a family meeting, and I was concerned because I had no idea how her mother was going to react. This was not going to be the first time she had heard her daughter's pain about that moment, and reports from previous programs never showed that any progress was made in this family's sessions. I admit, I was surprised by the exchange of emotions that occurred. Instead of guilt and accusations marking the first stage of the meeting, there were smiles and acceptance. While Janis's mother tried to bring up that event to defend herself again, Janis held up her hand to stop her. Then she said, "That moment has passed. I love both of you and that is enough. I want to count on you to help me get on with my life now. Will you help me find a life that I can be proud of, so I can like who I am and we can be a loving family again?" This was similar to a statement of forgiveness, in that Janis had found resolution within herself. Everyone rejoiced at the outcome of Janis's family session. Janis made plans to return to college in order to become a psychologist. Hope had returned.

When another person has harmed and wronged you, it is pretty rare to be able to confront them and receive an apology or expression of remorse. Your resolution is not likely to come from engaging that person at all. It's much more powerful to arrive at peace within, but reaching that state takes much time, inner reflection, and infusion with your personal wisdom. Like Janis, until we arrive at inner resolution, the person can continue to exert power over us and harm us—especially when we are so furious at them we become blind to how our actions actually hurt us. Resolution is a deeply personal journey that involves many steps and stages. I want you to know that it is possible, so keep to your path of healing and allow the rhythms of your being to support you.

MOVING FROM PAIN TO PURPOSE

The ongoing nature of trauma pain has been traced to a region deep in the brain called the *amygdala,* which records memories related to painful experiences—especially emotional pain. This may serve a survival purpose so we can learn what is dangerous to prevent—or not repeat—the same experience in the future. Brain mapping reveals that our tissues show increasing growth when a person or animal responds to past memories. In animals, certain medications can manage those fears and emotional reactions, but the drugs are dangerous to humans. I have found that, because musical rhythms have been shown to decrease the responses related to the amygdala and can treat PTSD and other traumas, it may be our most powerful treatment. It was this data that encouraged me to develop the BAUD.

The effectiveness of using the BAUD, as I did for Pete and Janis, likely results from the way it appears to cut short the neurological pattern that serves as a bridge through the looping thoughts of trauma. It helps us see past the fixations that constantly throw up stress barriers, which ring throughout our nervous system to cause imbalance. Using the metaphor of a car, fears and painful emotions would be like a dysfunction in the carburetor that causes the engine to backfire loudly. But when reset to a normal rhythm, it runs smoothly. Biofeedback technology, like the BAUD, allow for rhythmic balance of life demands to occur that include envisioning goals for our future and planning the steps that will get us there.

My favorite quote from Mark Twain is, *"The two most important days of your life are the day you were born and the day you find out why."* Sometimes it takes a loss of balance to inspire us to ask the profound question, *"Why am I here?"* Perhaps this is why painful experiences like trauma are included in earthly experience. It's the return to the rhythms of life, through the healing process, that helps us find meaning and fulfill our purpose.

PART III

ENCOURAGING WELLNESS IN OTHERS

So far in this book, I have shared insights into personal healing. By reading stories of suffering and resetting wellness, my hope is that you can now perceive the natural rhythms essential to healthy life patterns. Now I'd like to shift and share how you can apply healing rhythms to helping others. Whether you are a practitioner at a clinic or someone who wants to integrate a protocol of balance into your family's life, this part of *Healing Rhythms to Reset Wellness* is for you.

Supporting the body's rhythms in a practical, ongoing way involves a "wellness model" rather than the "illness model" most of us were educated in or grew up with. A wellness model consists of the practices and activities that reset our natural rhythms of health. It is a program of lifestyle changes that will bring us back to health and a protocol of practices that can be taught and shared.

I first became interested in the creation of wellness models when a team I led was tasked with combating the stress crisis in Japan. The objective, to put it bluntly, was to teach workers stress management skills, so they would not die from the stress of work demands. The insurance company tasked me with helping these individuals maintain a good quality of life without diminishing their health with disease and the limitations of chronic illness through their productive years as workers.

At first, I was surprised that my focus was not to be the younger workers. When we are young, wellness protocols can be preventative, so I naturally thought this would be the best place to start. But from the perspective of the economic investment of time and money, it made sense that the insurance company was prioritizing the older workers because, due to their years of work experience, they were the greatest investment. They were also under the greatest threat for chronic disease, cardiovascular syndromes, and chronic pain. When we are older, wellness protocols can facilitate more adaptive responses in us, which in turn, can help our bodies work with the changes and limitations of age, rather than resist them or buckle under them.

Along with the responsibility of training the staff, I consulted on the designing and building of instruments that measured change in the workers' behaviors; these instruments were used to measure their degree of mental health or mental illness. After five years of effort and success in Japan, I felt my time with the company needed to end. I departed with a sense of pride, feeling that I had effected change in the culture there.

At the same time, as I was pulling away from that work, I designed and created the first master's degree in behavioral medicine, which seeks to offer ways we can apply behaviors and lifestyle choices—rather than pills—in order to create change in our body-mind systems that promote balance and health. The curriculum included courses that are essential to the topic of wellness from many angles: psychological, physical, nutritional. It was a popular course from the start for one seemingly simple reason: it offered a *pragmatic* way to view life change in a broader context, taking all aspects of behavior into consideration, rather than attempting to perform quick fixes.

Aside from the intuitive and relatable ways that my master's wellness program landed with people, it was also popular because it did not shy away from the importance of considering the practicality, even on a national scale, of wellness behaviors. In America alone, industries and businesses spends over $300 billion on stress-related ailments and sick days every year. When someone gets sick, it costs their employer money. But what if, instead of paying for sick time and hospital costs, businesses prevented most of these costs? What if they supported healthy lifestyles, rather than paying to treat the outcome of unhealthy ones? They would use their funds to help prevent sickness, rather than react to it.

Although you may not be thinking of society as a whole when helping an individual patient or loved one, it is important to remember that wellness behaviors benefit more than just individuals—they concretely benefit businesses and bottom lines. So if you are a healer, doctor, or wellness practitioner, wellness programs are a smart investment. Not only are they not costly to implement, but I can't tell you how rewarding helping people or making these changes for your family can be. Participants usually design their own programs and hold themselves accountable. They rely on your mentorship and the education and encouragement you can give them. To put it simply: the investment pays for itself, as is not costly to implement.

A personalized wellness program could include an unlimited amount of new behaviors. But the list can be narrowed down with a focus on the areas of life, or symptoms, that are clamoring the loudest for attention. There are six areas I have found to be the easiest to access through rhythms. In the following chapters, I will bring each of these skills to life and make them accessible so you can help others implement them in their lives. My thoughts are based on my experiences in Japan, the thousands of patients I have supported, and the years of research I have invested in my essential desire to help others reset their rhythms for wellness.

CHAPTER 8

EASE STRESS

Don't give in to your fears. If you do, you won't be able
to talk to your heart.
–Paulo Coelho

At the top of a personal list of life problems often sits the word *stress*. Stress is a common, even universal, complaint. It can quickly disable the body's powerful restorative systems, causing a litany of further issues and complaints. This is why stress management needs to be a foundational component of any wellness concept and every wellness protocol. It is a core rhythmic conflict.

Although stress may strike us as a confusing cloud of feelings and sensations, it can be seen simply as an irregularity of rhythms within us. This "irregularity" promotes internal friction, conflict, and loss of energy. The disruptions causing this irregularity can occur from within, as well as from outside us. Every system of stress management—and there are many— aims to disrupt the irregularity and reset our rhythms so they can return to their natural pace once more.

Every stress-management system has its champions and its critics based on their personal preferences and experiences of efficacy. Meditation techniques, for example, are wonderful, but for some they are mysterious. They strike many in western culture as "boring." Some may think meditation is scary or off-limits because of beliefs about Eastern religions. If this is the case, find a meditation system that is stripped down to the essential, underlying principle—breathing—so it does not create friction for you or the person you are trying to support.

Here are my recommendations for a variety of systems that you or the person you are supporting can choose between. Consider what you have heard works for others or what has worked for you. Someone may have had a good or bad experience with one or two methods of stress management, and that is okay; there is a plentiful menu of wonderful options to choose from.

THE EMWAVE2 DEVICE (WWW.HEARTMATH.ORG)

The EmWave2 device is a personal biofeedback device. It is the most technical of my recommendations, but it is also the quickest to learn. This device is the size of a package of gum and utilizes a sophisticated computer with complex algorithms that calculate the appropriate breathing pattern to bring you into balance.

The Protocol
The participant turns it on and attaches an ear clip or places their thumb on the red region of the device.

- During the first stage, it reads the participant's heart rate variability, which is a measure of stress. This takes about ten seconds.

- During the second stage, a light bar appears and prompts a particular breathing pattern in the participant. Their breathing is being re-trained as they sync its rhythm with the light.

- During the third stage, a biofeedback light flashes red, blue, or green to show the participant when they are breathing correctly (red means "not correct," blue and green means "correct"). These signals are also interpreted as "points," thus offering the participant a sense of reward, which can be helpful reinforcement in the re-training process.

I have found this approach most successful when I use the red light to counter the stress signals by retraining my brain focus using the breathing pattern toward the green light (Alab-dulgader, 2012; Peavey, 1985).

BAUD: BIO-ACOUSTICAL UTILIZATION DEVICE (WWW.BAUDENERGETICS.COM)

This device is most effective when the stress being treated by it is related to a specific event or trauma that interferes with the basic emotional rhythms of peace and joy. It is also excellent for disrupting patterns of anxious thinking.

The Protocol

As I showed you through case studies in Part II of this book, the BAUD method isolates the stress frequency, which can be any stress-inducing state, even physical pain. It does so by having the participant use a pitch knob in order to increase the stressful feeling. When you feel stressed, you know you've found the right frequency.

The second step is then to disrupt that frequency with the disruptor knob. It sounds quick, and it certainly can be, but it may take some time. Finding a frequency that increases joy, rather than one that increases stress, is also effective. Either way, the goal is to locate a frequency that affects the participant's neural rhythms immediately, either disrupting the ones that need to be changed or enhancing the ones that are more desirable (Miller, 2017).

SENSORY DEPRIVATION CHAMBER

Sensory deprivation chambers hold huge appeal for people because of the peaceful state they can achieve inside them. Because the concept is simple—people almost intuitively feel such an experience would be a relief to their stress—it is a very accessible option.

The Protocol

Instruct the participant to lie down and relax. You can remind them that the sudden removal of outside stimulus may trigger a heightened awareness of their thoughts or concerns. Remind them that this is natural. This process can be accompanied with relaxing music. In a study observing over three thousand patients, the results of the thoughtful use of sensory deprivation chambers were consistently positive (Kjellgren, 2014).

HEALING SOUNDS

The website www.mindbodybylawlis.com provides affordable downloads, each of which have their own properties for stress management. Each soundtrack can be seen as a different medicine, taken for a different stress type. The following are some of my favorites:

*   *Homeostasis*—This soundtrack harmonizes the mind and body and simplifies life struggles in order to support the resetting of priorities. It also supports existential insight in order to help clarify personal missions.

*   *Neurological Stimulation for Joy*—This soundtrack stimulates energy, combats sadness, and inspires the listener to move more joyously throughout their day.

*   *Awakening*—This soundtrack increases mental creativity and problem-solving and stimulates intellectual pursuits.

*   *Gonging*—This soundtrack arrests looping thoughts, like obsessive thinking or worrying. It also increases attention span and the listener's experience of brain control.

- *Heartbeat Rhythm*—This soundtrack induces deep states of sleep and restores depleted energy (Thoma, 2013).

BREATHING TRAINING

Any breathing technique can be adjusted to the personal goals of the stressed person looking to reset their wellness rhythms. Sometimes breathing techniques are used with the goal of purification or simplification of thought, and sometimes they are used for relaxation.

The Protocol

- Music and breath—The *Relaxation with Flute* soundtrack from MindbodybyLawlis.com is a training soundtrack that includes breath and music. It helps participants relax and sometimes even fall asleep.

- Alternate nostril breathing—Closing one and then the other nostril with a finger pressed on the outside of the nostril, and breathing alternately through each nostril, supports the reduction of anger and rage. It also increases focus and concentration in participants.

- Stretch breath—Stretch breathing is breathing in to a count of 7 and out to a count of 7 in long, slow, deep, relaxed breaths. This practice forces participants to slow down, relax, and become more aware of the present moment.

- The "3-5-7" Exercise—Breathe in for a count of 3, hold for a count of 5, and exhale for a count of 7. This technique supports anxiety relief, relaxation, and calm. It also increases focus (Publishing, 2015).

EXERCISE

There are many good reasons to exercise. From a stress-management perspective, the foundational purpose of exercise is to help us energetically realign our muscles, body tissues, and organs. Raising energy levels creates a heightened coordination among the various rhythms that move our bodies. Heightened coordination in us automatically increases the vitality of our neural system, especially the cerebellum. Most importantly, perhaps, when we exercise we feel a whole lot better—unless exercise is overdone, of course. Simply put, exercise is a healthy and easy way to reduce stress effectively.

The Protocol

We should all be doing one of the following activities for at least twenty minutes a day. Consider that the standard time—twenty minutes for most people—must take into consideration any age and any inflammation issues that may be present.

- Yoga and Tai Chi

- Running, walking, hiking

- Dancing

- Sports and weight training (America, n.d.)

AROMAS

Aromas are potent agents for changing a mood, and a change in mood can mean a shift in rhythms. Aromas are also individualized—a pleasing aroma for one person can be abhorrent to another. The easiest way to use aroma is with essential oils, which are natural oils that hold the fragrance of the plant from which they were extracted. Some can be applied topically, some can be added to baths, and some can be diffused into the air. Encourage experimentation and play—there are so many aromas to play with, and it is easy to personalize essential oils as part of a wellness protocol (Kandhasamy Sowndhararajan, 2016).

MEDITATION

There are many excellent meditation methods, including scientifically developed ones, so you can choose a system or systems that the person you are supporting is most responsive to. Meditation can play an effective role in stress management, but what is meant by the term *meditation* seems to vary greatly. There are huge differences in how many of us define this seemingly simple activity. There are as many different strategies as there are instructors, it seems. In an effort to clarify the topic, I want to share three categories of meditation experiences. Each has its own power and purpose. Probably the most technical types are the most trustworthy, although most of them can be boiled down to one underlying focus—breathing.

"Alpha" meditation is any meditation practice in which we are learning to focus, moment-by-moment, on what is happening around and/or within us. I call it *Alpha* because it summons the relaxation level of the brain, thus distracting us from irrelevant worries and stressors. By deliberately focusing on what is happening now, we can access the reality of what is occurring in the present as the only thing that is "real." I see this important lesson as a valid reality check for those suffering from the irregular rhythms of anxiety.

"Theta" meditation allows us to practice being aware of multiple realities at once, which can be a helpful way of imagining the symbols and experiences of life in a new way. For example, one can imagine going on a journey and visiting multiple possibilities. When practiced in service of decision-making, Theta meditations can allow us to "have a foot in each world" and experience the wisdom and consequences of options before acting. Human beings appear to have this ability uniquely—to project our minds into the future in this way. For me, it is easier to practice Theta meditation accompanied by a drum beat in the theta frequency— four to five beats per second. This version of meditation is helpful for decision-making and envisioning new ways of being.

"Delta" meditation helps us practice "emptying" our minds of all activity and concerns. For me, this is very difficult, so perhaps I am not the best to judge of its benefits. Delta meditation takes discipline. Instruction in this technique is essential, which can be a barrier, but

I see good results from those who practice it. Practitioners say they are better able to know their own minds and patterns of thought when they practice it regularly (Laboratory, 2018).

IMAGERY FOR EMPOWERMENT AND RELAXATION

Imagery is the language of the brain. Empowering imagery helps us visualize ourselves and our attributes in new and interesting ways. Such imagery boosts our confidence and can introduce us to positive traits in ourselves that we may not have known about or have been utilizing. Relaxing imagery sends messages of peace and calm throughout the entire mind and thus, the body. This imagination play creates the opportunity for distress to give way to relaxation and it lowers blood pressure (Nguyen, 2018).

Protocol for Empowerment: Many top athletes have described this kind of empowering imagination play to be a source of ultra-human potential (King, 2010). The practice of it can look like imagining that you are an animal or a tree—anything that possesses qualities you are looking to embody.

Protocol for Relaxation: Relaxation imagery invites you to imagine yourself in a place in nature where you feel totally safe, secure, and at ease—a swing you loved at your grandparents' house when you were a child or the perfect beach you visited on vacation. It may also be a setting that comes purely from your imagination, with no tie to the physical world. It is a place you feel good, perhaps even the best.

These ideas are all well-respected and effective protocols for stress management and reduction. I have seen many of them, when practiced diligently, transform people's lives. Even in a fast-paced, demanding world, we can meet today's challenges by training to strengthen our ability to relax. No one needs to seesaw between hyperactivity and collapse when they know how to reset the balance of wellness.

CHAPTER 9

BOOST NUTRITION

Our bodies are our gardens; our wills are our gardeners.
—William Shakespeare

Of all the classes in my master's program on wellness, the class on nutrition is always the most well-attended. A contemplation on nutrition certainly belongs in any study of rhythms and health. Along with sleep, food is a naturally cycling part of each of our days. We eat, we are satiated, we do other activities until we are hungry, and we eat again. We give a lot of attention to the life rhythm of putting food in our body, sometimes worrying if we ate the right food and if it is adding to or subtracting from our well-being, and then monitoring how it comes out on the other end. Unwanted weight and constipation are often talked about topics—sometimes even with strangers—because these two areas often hold a lot of information about the state of our health and our quality of life.

Our emotions tend to overwhelm our cycle of nutrition, both internally and externally. Emotions may, and often do, determine what food we reach for throughout our day.

Internally, our emotional state also plays into how we digest our food. Studies have shown, for example, that the amount of food we eat during a meal is surprisingly unrelated to how full we feel during that meal. One factor leading to obesity and anorexia is overriding or denying our stomach's capacity based on messages from our metabolic system. Another factor is listening to the psychological messages we say to ourselves about what we "need" to eat based on our programmed minds. Our pleasure centers can reach the point of addiction to certain foods and in doing so, can override healthy rhythms.

Our relationship with nutrition likely began in the kitchen, around the dinner table, or in front of the TV—in the circumstances and family dynamics that surrounded food in our childhoods. The power of the dinner table is often romanticized in our culture, but the overriding anxiety that is so often present in such family settings can lead to obsession and damage around food and family relationships throughout life. Suffering that began at the dinner table can then be further amplified by the unrealistic models of beauty that girls and boys compare themselves to. Eating disorders are the consequences of such anxieties. Fear of looking "unattractive" in our culture, even into adulthood, alters what we eat and how much we eat.

In youth, our metabolism reigns mighty, sometimes despite our emotionally driven nutritional choices, but age catches up quickly. Without external safeguards to monitor what we eat and how high quality it is, it is no wonder we are an obese nation. Health insurance companies have discovered that weight issues are directly tied to chronic disease and have begun to consider this connection in their premiums. Employers have also correlated weight issues with work performance and thus, sometimes consider weight in their hiring policies. Such biases may be unfair, as genetics *do* play a part when it comes to weight, but it is now a reality that obesity is economically punished.

We owe it to ourselves to reset our metabolisms back to healthy patterns because we can. No weight loss pill or surgery can save anyone from themselves; we have to educate ourselves and others and behave our way back to a healthy rhythm of nutrition. That is a central part of the mission of this wellness program.

THE MIND RESET: DON'T TRUST YOUR BODY

As odd as it sounds, "don't trust your body" is a key first step in resetting the body's rhythm around food. It is important to understand that the fat developed by the body begins to have a life of its own. It actually develops its own hormone system that then creates its own defense system that then sabotages our motivation to trim it off. Furthermore, the hormone *ghrelin*, which signals to us that we have reached that "full" feeling, gets turned off. On top of that, the signals from the waist "stretch cells" minimize their signals as well. Now, with the physical cues gone that were so important in knowing when to stop, we are only as strong as our self-control. This situation is like flying an airplane in total darkness without any instruments. Sooner or later, your sense of balance will cause you to overcorrect the controls and you will spin the plane to your demise. Sadly, the effects of weight gain can really be this dire for many of us.

The reality of what it takes to balance your nutrition, or to help a patient or loved one do the same, is this: deny your emotions and hunger signals completely. Begin to rely instead on visual cues and your intelligence when making food choices. The following are rules that I know will help implement this mind reset and regain healthy nutritional rhythms.

RESET NUTRITIONAL RHYTHMS

When working toward a reset of nutritional rhythms, take on one thing at a time. Don't overwhelm yourself or the person who you are trying to support by trying to do it all at once or demanding that they do so. That is a recipe for failure. For instance, if sugar is the craving, start reducing the intake of sugar, one snack or meal at a time. Instead of eating a candy bar, eat an orange. Instead of drinking a soda, drink coffee or tea. Substitute one rhythm at a time. Don't stop eating the wrong food at first, instead substitute it for something else. You can also try, or recommend, replacing a particular food rhythm with exercise. If someone cyclically craves sugar after work, they should try taking a nice long walk. A walk will provide almost the same biochemical responses as the sugar would have (Hills, 2013).

EAT BY THE CLOCK

This rule invites us to be consistent about when we eat. If you feel you have good energy throughout the day from eating at 7:30 a.m., noon, and 6:00 p.m., eat consistently during those times. If you are helping someone who is not a breakfast eater and thrives on only two meals a day, then help them plan accordingly. If someone eats ten small snacks a day, then they should be consistent with that plan. Each of us should explore what works for us, then do that every day.

Unfortunately, there is no magic system that fits everyone. One's personal rhythm processes food according to one's needs. One's personal rhythm primes the metabolism to adjust when it needs to, but only if it knows when it needs to do so. This is the reason that fasting does not work. If we withhold food from our body at a time it is used to receiving food, it will store it. Then, when food finally does come along, the body will promptly turn that food into fat because it doesn't want us to starve. If we develop the very unhealthy habit of purging after each meal, the same thing will happen.

To accomplish this process with your body or to support someone else doing the same, start paying attention to energy levels throughout the day and begin to experiment with the pace of energy flow that eating certain foods at certain times provides. Teach your patient or loved one to stop themselves from eating when they are upset, stressed, or bored—usually, these moods fall outside the times when they would be routinely eating, anyway. Our adrenals typically raise in intensity of activity during the late morning and gradually fall in the afternoon and into the evening. That being said, our natural metabolic schedules can easily be shifted by circumstance, so encourage your patient or loved one to pay attention to what is happening for them. Perhaps their job only allows them to eat at specific times, but that's okay—their body will comply to the consistency. It takes about six weeks to develop a habit; interestingly, it takes a similar time period for our metabolisms to adapt as well (Council, 2019).

OBJECTIVELY JUDGE YOUR FOOD

Instruct your patient or loved one to turn their focus away from judgment of what others eat, or perhaps jealousy over what they can "get away with," and instead, pay attention to their own needs. Help educate them as to what foods are essential in creating a healthy rhythm of metabolism *for them*. At last count, I believe I have seen 1,004 diets out there that guarantee perfect health, if only one follows some "expert's" plan.

Calorie-counting is not the answer either because there are good calories and bad calories. Let me explain why: Calories are the heat a food produces when it is burned up. There is some correlation to the nature of how it is metabolized in the human body, but such a system has nothing to do with our personal process when we eat food, use it, and then dispose of it.

FOLLOW A FOOD PROTOCOL

In Chapter 3, I have offered a food plan, but here is the protocol in its simplest form for those of you wanting to help yourself, those you care for at work, or those at home make these changes.

- ◆ Avoid sugar, salt, and preservatives

- ◆ Eat protein and complex carbonates

- ◆ Eat nuts

- ◆ Eat fresh vegetables

- Eat fresh fruit with skins or leaves

- In the preparation of food, eat the rawest and healthiest version of whatever you take. The more heat you put your food through, the more difficult it is for your body to recognize it as food. When heat is applied to food, its molecular structure is changed. A raw egg, for example, maximizes your metabolism; a boiled egg is helpful to your body in a reduced way; a fried egg is the worst! The heating and frying process is what creates the cholesterol that harms your heart. A French fry is no longer a potato, nor is it a potato chip.

- Avoid additives and processed food. If our bodies do not recognize something as food, then it is experienced by our bodies as garbage. The body has to deal with that garbage before it can digest the good stuff. In these moments, the rhythm of the metabolism is slowed, disrupted, or even halted.

- Care about your elimination! With the same concept of the rhythms of our body's metabolism, I recommend foods that assist in healthy, rhythmic elimination. Unless there is a consistent process of elimination, the body has to deal with the toxicities of the used food and poisons can accumulate in your system. Here are the foods on the anti-constipation list:

Liquids: water, coffee, tea, lemon juice, apple cider vinegar

Fruits and vegetables: spinach, oranges, strawberries with leaves, prunes, pears, broccoli, carrots, peaches, pineapple, figs

Beans, nuts, and flaxseeds

Yogurt

Cumin

Magnesium (Crosby, 2016)

CONTROL YOUR CRAVINGS

The body creates cravings for certain foods; sugary and salty foods are often high on that craving list. Such cravings can easily lead to a lifestyle that seriously hampers proper food rhythms because we frequently get sidetracked by snacks. When snack after snack of sugary foods is eaten, the insulin production in the pancreas gets wrecked. In order for the body to metabolize food, especially sugar, insulin has to be produced and fed into the system as a carrier of the food cells. But if the insulin production is not secreted in direct relationship to the intake of food, or if the rhythms are not regular, the cells get stressed and eventually become unusable or resistant. Sometimes they disappear completely. The former outcome is type 2 diabetes, and the latter is type 1 diabetes.

I know of only two ways to control these cravings. One is the BAUD system. To support the elimination of cravings, the participant sets the pitch frequency to relate to the imagery of the problem food and the disruptor knob to the feeling that the craving is gone. The BAUD system locates a frequency that effects the neural rhythms associated with the craving and disrupts the strength of the habit-loop the participant's brain is in around these unhealthy foods. I have personally observed this system to work on the cessation of cravings for French fries, chocolate, cookies, soda, ice cream, and pure processed sugar.

The second way to control cravings it is to go cold turkey. Every time the image of the food they are craving comes up, the person seeking relief should relax and do some deep breathing. Aromatherapy can also really help, as it disrupts the neuro-logical signals of the craving (Myers, 2018). Cold turkey is certainly not an easy approach, but sometimes the boundary it offers can be immensely supportive to those in craving distress.

COUNT YOUR CHEWS

It is not just a myth that the more we chew our food, the better it is for us. First of all, broken-down food is easier to absorb. Second, the meal takes longer when we chew it and we then eat less of the food. Third, chewing our food helps the rhythms of digestion because the organs further down the digestive chain are able to work at their best when they receive well broken-down food. The question is: how long does one chew? My estimate, depending on the kind of food being consumed, is that thirty chews is a good average. By the way, such activity also allows more time for others at the table to talk, which is usually appreciated (Farooq, 2016).

DIVIDE THE MEAL IN HALF AND SAVE HALF FOR LATER

This advice does not mean that we should make or order a bigger meal to begin with. Start with an average-sized plate. Ordinarily, this size would be what we get when ordering from a restaurant, but the fast-food businesses often make king-sized portions, especially of the wrong foods (D., 2015). Again, train yourself or the person you are supporting to use visual judgments about the portion, rather than emotional or feeling-based ones. Your client might be surprised how energized they feel when taking in a bit less food during one sitting.

Nutrition is a big topic in today's world. We eat too much, we throw away too much, and we don't allow our metabolisms to serve us well. For the first time in history, we have to be taught how to manage our food for our best functioning. Luckily, managing our nutrition can be learned and practiced. The body's digestive rhythms can be extremely powerful, if we don't make their job harder than it needs to be.

CHAPTER 10

ENJOY MOVEMENT

What you get by achieving your goals is not as important as what you become.
–Zig Ziglar

Do you remember getting your first bicycle or ballet slippers? What about a hula hoop or a baseball glove? As children, the "toys" that surrounded exercise were some of the most exciting. But besides that, the wind in our hair, the camaraderie on the field, and the simple joy of movement for movement's sake, also made exercise a carefree part of our days. Though we are adults now, we can still get excited about barbells and bicycles; this is why exercise and movement are probably the most commonly used methods in wellness programs. The simple facts back this up—exercise has so many excellent health benefits for us. Movement returns us to those happy days when exercise was not a task we had to check of our to-do list; it was a part of the fabric of our lives and how we moved around the world. Playful fun, not efficiency, was our movement goal.

Unless physical movement was disrupted for us in some way as a child, the perception that exercise can be fun is fortunate because we can tap back into this early experience of exercise equaling fun when helping others or ourselves. This is important because movement may be the single most important part of wellness rhythms.

OUR EXERCISE NEEDS CHANGE OVER TIME

Movement is especially essential for those with "executive" jobs—those who work long hours at a desk that is littered with papers and responsibilities. Meet Thomas, a prime example of an executive for whom exercise became a crucial and life-changing part of his wellness protocol over many decades of his life. His needs and challenges evolved as he aged, but the themes remained the same.

When Thomas was in his earlies twenties, he was recruited from an elite program at Texas Tech. His academic background was a blend of computer technology, programming, and hardware. He was noticeably skilled at resolving complaints from customers. He was creative and had a likable personality, so he soared in his job assignments interpersonally, while also busting through the front lines of development of sophisticated and sellable software systems. Thomas was going like gangbusters.

The only hitch? Thomas loved his work so much that he spent late hours at his desk, contemplating work problems. Did this result in bonuses and increases at work? Of course. But at the same time, due to the stress and physical stillness, his body was aging rapidly. He was losing weight and muscle mass, which was resulting in the loss of his rhythmic energy.

When Thomas first came to me, it was apparent that the best thing he could do for himself was to schedule time five days a week, during the day or evening, to exercise in a way that he enjoyed. I invited him to see these times as appointments with himself. He needed to make these appointments as much of a priority as he would have if they had been with his CEO and not his bicycle. There was nothing more important, I pointed out to him.

Thomas embraced his wellness program happily, quickly remembering that he enjoyed cycling, and that new technology would allow him to do live classes from stationary bikes he moved into his home and his office. He also made a repetitive weight-lifting schedule a part of his new routine. The extended endurance these types of movements gave him quickly made an impact on his endurance at work as well. At the end of each of his "movement appointments" with himself, Thomas would relax and allow his mind to move into a Theta state. By letting his brain meditate on the frequency that heightens creativity and restoration, Thomas was also bringing his mind back toward the rhythms of his naturally creative personality. Thomas's new wellness routine worked. His muscle tone came back, and so did his momentum and stamina at work. He felt less burnt out at the end of his days and more connected to himself than he had before.

But time progressed and, as is the case for many of us, other priorities began to interfere and crowd out Thomas's time. He married his high school sweetheart, had three children, and bought a house. The house was a little beyond his means, but with his job success, he was confident that the purchase was sound. He was promoted through the ranks, changing companies on his way up the ladder. He nailed goal after goal. The only bump in his journey of success was the time he skipped a conference he should have attended for work in order to compete in a bike race. Having seen the effects of not prioritizing work, he resolved the issue by demonstrating his devotion to his work obligations and let competitive sports take a backseat.

By the time he was in his late forties, Thomas was the vice president of a large company. He was highly admired for his work ethic as well as his creativity, but he spent fifty-five hours a week, once again, sitting at his desk and neglecting the physical rhythms necessary for the intense demands of his position and duties. His heart was beating in irregular paces, the muscles in his lower back (the lumbar region) were highly imbalanced. Every day, the muscle spasms in his back got more intense. He was overweight by eighty pounds. He was taking anti-anxiety medications to deal with the stress of his work and he was taking opioid pain pills to deal with the pain in his back. He was forty-seven, but he looked like he was sixty-seven. Worse, he later told me he had felt even older than sixty-seven at the time.

It had been years since I had last seen Thomas when he reappeared one day at my wellness center. He didn't want to get back surgery, he said, and coming to me was his effort to reclaim his wellness again, as he had all those years before. He hoped that, by restarting his concert of rhythms, he would soon access a better state of health.

Once again, we focused on exercise and stress-relief elements, modified in service of his age and needs. Instead of the theta meditation, he selected the delta meditation. Theta meditation had been to increase the creative-flow states in his brain, but he knew that what he needed now was delta meditation because he needed a parasympathetic focus for his health. The fact that he was on anti-anxiety medication was also a clue that he needed restorative practices, not stimulating ones.

Sleep had been increasingly difficult for Thomas, and he knew he needed to restore the rhythmic balance of that essential nightly reset. The new exercise program we designed for him combined core body strengthening (exercises aimed at supporting the back, abdominal, and pelvic muscles), cardiovascular training (exercises aimed at supporting one's breathing and heart-rate endurance), and exercises aimed at supporting his realignment and balance. Thomas also asked for a nutritional program to help shift off his extra pounds and leave him with more energy to face his busy life.

Thomas's story is one of renewal, from many perspectives. Being a highly disciplined person by nature, he regained his body rhythms back within three months' time. His heart rhythms and blood pressure became normal again and his back pain subsided to the point that he was able to stop taking pain medication. His weight was on the downward slide; after three months, he had lost about forty pounds. What health practitioners would call Thomas's "metrics," like weight and blood pressure, were all now within what are considered normal, healthy limits.

But the psychological changes in Thomas were even more remarkable and thrilling to watch unfold. Thomas's life was now balanced such that he and his family enjoyed time and space together, now that Thomas was not consumed by work 24/7. Thomas became a better, more attentive partner. He now had the mental space to use his talent for conflict resolution at home, not just at work, and thus there was much less domestic turmoil. His outlook on life began to extend beyond just his career and social power. By recommitting to himself once again, as he had those many years ago, I noticed that Thomas was now spending more time demonstrating his love for others and less time focusing on himself. His commitment to his wellness continued into other realms of contentment as well. He even missed a conference or two in favor of a passion of his that had previously been set aside: to make a difference in world hunger. He served as a volunteer in the World Health Organization and helped create effective sewer systems in Africa. Thomas' life became an inspirational one, a life well-lived.

WEAVING EXERCISE AND MOVEMENT INTO LIFE

Thomas's journey shows us that there are at least three ways we can approach exercise as part of a wellness model. These three approaches—or doorways—are endurance exercise, core building, and recreational movement. When designing a wellness protocol for yourself or someone else, consider which of these areas is most needed in the participant's life. Also keep in mind the importance of including all three, in some way.

Endurance Exercises: These use repetitive power movements that build physical endurance. The goal is to add to the reserve of energy in the body. One of the basic versions of this in a wellness protocol is an exercise in which the participant lifts a ten-pound barbell twenty times or more. Or perhaps they press (while laying on their back and pushing upward) the barbell twenty times at first. Later, the participant can begin to push for a higher numbers of times as the new goal. If one were doing this as an endurance exercise, one would not increase the weight, only the number of repetitions. Stamina—not muscle growth—is the goal here. A similar strategy would apply to building one's leg endurance. One exercise might be lifting a small weight twenty times at first, with the goal of increasing the repetitions count later. Bicycling goals would be set to the number of miles ridden, although the advantage of the bicycle would be the opportunity to vary the demands of the journey with uphill and downhill runs. Again, the view of the "endurance" approach is to improve cardiovascular endurance and the muscle mass needed to carry out those cardiovascular-supporting activities.

Core Strength: When we have strength in the inner body—the abdominals, the back, the chest, the neck—we are less likely to be injured and more likely to feel at home in our own bodies. I find it safer to use weight machines, the kind in the local gym, to locate these muscle groups, although free weights have an advantage in that they demand our coordination and stabilization, which in turn, improves our internal rhythm and balance. When core strength is the goal, the protocol is to increase the weight lifted or pushed in five repetitions at a time as our tissues grow in power and ability.

Recreational Movement: The goal here is to feel the sheer joy of motion. This can look like dancing, jumping on a trampoline, or taking a martial art. Singing can also tune us into the pulsing rhythms in our bodies. There is rhythmic music in all of us that is always available for us to move to and move with. Recreational movement has the added benefit of helping us access joints and smaller muscles we may not be using so much during our habitual gym or cardio routines. Recreational movement is also well-suited to those of us whose strengths and flexibilities are limited, such as the elderly, people in wheelchairs, or those who are missing limbs or lack full control of theirs. These types of lively and very human forms of movement do not discriminate on the basis of age or physical and cognitive functioning. Recreational movement can also easily begin to build our endurance, perhaps without us even noticing.

STRETCHING IS NATURAL

While animals do not use weights or machines to maintain their muscular rhythmic health, they *do* use stretching. Animals will stretch after a length of time spent in stillness. They will yawn and shake their heads. When we under-use our muscles, we shorten them. If we spend a lot of our time sitting at a desk, we are shortening one set of our muscles and not shortening the opposing muscles. This imbalance will lead to unusual pressures on the joints and lead to inflammation. These days, this is a common problem.

The protocol is simple, but consistency can take some practice. You, or the person you are helping, must be educated about stretching each set of the body's muscles in the following manner. My advice is to put a stretch on the muscle group to the point of tension without pain. Then hold the stretch until it releases further, while breathing deeply. There is no need or point in pumping the muscle—just stretch and hold while relaxing that muscle group, thus allowing the limb to relax and release further.

The muscle groups that are usually the most prone to stress, and thus need to be regularly stretched, are as follows. Follow this routine daily, or even multiple times a day, and invite those you are supporting in their wellness to do so as well.

Stretching the Traps

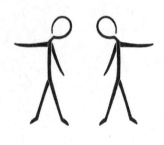

The **traps** are located between the shoulder and the head. To stretch the right side of the body, extend the right arm out to the side while tilting the head to the left. For the left side, extend the left arm to the side while tilting the head to the right.

Stretching the Neck

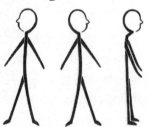

To stretch the **neck,** gently twist the head to the left, then stretch and turn the head to the right. Then gently press the head forward while holding the chin up.

Stretching the Back

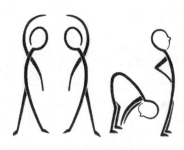

To stretch the **back** from the waist, raise the right arm overhead while stretching the back to the right. Reverse to the left. Now bend forward, stretching out the lower back muscles and bending backward with a stretch. Breathe and relax.

Stretching the Legs

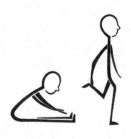

Here are two different ways to stretch the **legs**. While sitting, stretch the body forward, hinging from the hip. With each breath, reach for the toes. Or while standing, pull the right leg up behind the butt, stretching out the thigh muscles along the front. Then reverse the process with the other leg. Some may need a long belt or rope around the lifted foot in order to elevate it.

Stretching the Feet

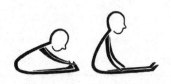

To stretch the **feet**, use a rope or belt around the feet, or use the hands if they can reach the feet. Pull the feet towards you, stretching the bottom muscle group. Then point your toes downward, away from you, for a stretch on the top of the foot.

Stretching the Hands

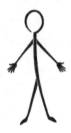

Perhaps surprisingly, your **hands** are very vulnerable to stress. Stretch your fingers and wrists in rhythm with your breath—flex them out as you breathe in and relax them as you breathe out.

These are basic stretches, but notice—or ask your patients and loved ones if they notice— feeling some rise in the body's heat when these stretches are done, maybe even to the point of a light sweat. This is normal, and a sign that our muscles are releasing the stress they have accumulated from the spasms and lactic acid that builds up in them when we use them, or don't use them, and then fail to stretch. If you or someone you are helping would like to make stretching an even greater part of their wellness protocol, I also recommend tai chi and yoga.

POSTURES FOR EMOTIONAL RELEASE

Based on the philosophy of bioenergetics, a field of study that attends to the movement of energy within the body, and observations I have made about carvings in ancient temples, there is some indication that certain postures release emotional blockages. We can see these postures reflected in statues of famous people, indicating their message. Like different aromas can soothe different mental states, or different sound waves bring the mind out of different loops, so each of these postures can support different emotional needs. The following five postures empower a more rhythmic flow of energy in five areas of life (Jeanne Achterberg, 1980).

The Victory Posture

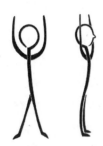

The **Victory Posture** is like one is celebrating something, except with minor differences. It is formed by raising the hands above the head, with the shoulders extended backward, exposing and bumping out the chest. The back is arched backward, with the knees slightly bent.

I have found that it is impossible for a person to assume this posture and feel depressed. If a person you are helping appears chronically sad and depressed, have him or her assume the Victory Posture for five minutes a day. It will be difficult for them—unnatural, even—but the results will likely be a pause in the emotional lock that is depression.

The Focus Posture

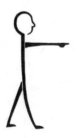

The **Focus Posture** is assumed by the participant standing with their dominant foot extended forward, along with their dominant hand directly before them. The index finger is pointed forward. All their energies and their eyes are directed forward. I use this posture with people with "motivation ambivalence," meaning they can't decide which direction they want to take. After five minutes, I invite them to notice how they felt about the decision they were stuck on while in this position—did they feel more strongly one way or the other? Again and again, I notice that assuming the Focus Posture helps people make decisions.

The Turtle Posture

The **Turtle Posture** is like self-cuddling! The body is curled up in a knot, with the legs tucked up under the body, as well as the hands and arms. The head is also tucked down between the shoulders. The Turtle Posture creates a sense of safety and protection. Sometimes a person is so stressed and vulnerable that this posture can offer the chance to withdraw. The downward, inward-facing focus can bring the attention to his or her needs at the present time. I have used this posture when a person is grieving over a loss. In this position, they are able to escape the pressure to pay attention to others and find a safe place to resolve some of their sadness with some privacy.

The Power Posture

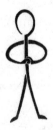

To assume the **Power Posture**, the participant creates a ring with their arms in front of them and makes a fist in the dominant hand and wraps that fist with the other hand. The eyes are directed straight ahead, with the chest muscles pressing the two hands together. You might recognize this posture from depictions throughout culture of warriors confronting their enemies. I have invited people to use this posture when preparing to confront a challenge (like a phone call with the IRS) and want to feel their power. Slogans can be recited while in this posture: *"I can handle this"* or *"I am powerful."*

The Healing Posture

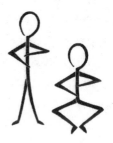

The **Healing Posture** is by far the most frequently seen posture in temples and ashrams. This posture is assumed by placing the left hand over the heart and the right hand over the belly button (or "Kath" chakra). The participant can sit or stand, but either way they should embody a meditative attitude and breath. Participants often notice a sudden rise in their body heat, as well as a rise in their internal body. The theory behind this posture is that energies are collected through the hands' energies. I believe that the immunities of the white blood cells are stimulated as well; people have reported to me that their sickness symptoms disappear when using this posture.

MOVING OURSELVES TOWARD RESET

Research is consistent in its report: Our bodies change through exercise and movement because these things stimulate rhythmic flow. The benefits of exercise have also been proven to increase our ability to learn, remember, and produce new nerve cells and brain cells. Exercise speeds up *neurotransmission*, which is the messaging system in our brains (Cotman, 2007). Movement positively affects the neurotransmitters in our brains: dopamine, noradrenaline, and serotonin. Thus, it reduces depression and anxiety and improves our resilience and ability to cope with whatever comes our way in life (Chaouloff, 1989).

The studies are important and helpful, but both the animal kingdom and human cultures have known the importance of physical movement for all of history. Movement and dance has been associated with rituals of healing performed for the gods, and movement and dance play a part in symbols of healing around the world. It is interesting that, while many of these rituals have a cleansing motive to them, most of them also call on divine strength for survival. Perhaps we can now call on and utilize the underlying, powerful rhythms of our biology to help ourselves and others heal through motion.

CHAPTER 11

BREAK ADDICTION

Between stimulus and response, there is a space. In the space
there is the power to choose our response. In our response
lies our growth and our freedom.
–Victor Frankl

My efforts to help people with addiction have revealed, most profoundly, that the best way to regain balanced life rhythms is through increasing hope and incorporating life skills. We tend to try to scare people into quitting a substance—think of all the smoking cessation efforts through ghastly images of jaws or noses missing and fifty-year-olds who look like ninety-year-olds. I too assumed that the scary messages must work in motivating people to stop the destructive behaviors of smoking, so I kept that in mind as I developed a "Stop Smoking" video in the mid-1980s.

I had been approached to collaborate on an effort out of New Zealand with the movie industry. Based on my reputation in the field of imagery, the firm had the idea for a video program. Their highest priority was a smoking-cessation project, along with a stress, weight, and cancer-management project they would launch later on. The vision was to integrate the visual animation and the verbal narration in the video such that the smoker viewer's brain would remain in an Alpha state—the state of creativity, imagination, and intuition—while being supported, somehow, in giving up cigarettes.

I was excited about this project for several reasons. Merging the wellness movement and the film industry into an experiential video to alter the brain frequencies of viewers at home was a new idea at the time. Projects like these take several trials. At each stage, the content is run by an audience and their response determines what gets adjusted before moving forward. During the first trial, the team needed to uncover what video images would induce a state of relaxation in the viewer. In spite of my expertise in the field of the relaxation of the conscious mind, I guessed wrong. I had figured that waterfalls, scenic sunsets, flowers blooming, and birds flying would induce relaxation—but no! We observed that all these images actually woke the brain up. The novelty of the scenes and the past memories they triggered activated the brain rather than relaxing it.

What were the images that did induce deep relaxation? They were images of extremely slow action and foggy images that did not look like real things. One image that worked well was that of a sailboat slowly passing from one side of the screen to the other over the span of about ten minutes. The other images that induced relaxation were of clouds slowly emerging around each other with no clear conceptual point, of ice breaking, and of colored drops falling into water and dispersing.

I had written scripts to go along with these images and they were read by a man with a low, seductive voice and British accent. I coached him on how to phrase the relaxation words in order to emphasize the power of our lesson. With the imagery and the voice in place, the next phase of the project was to try the video with real smokers who wanted to quit. You can imagine my shock when the video ended and they got up from their chairs, turned off the monitor, and lit up a cigarette. The video did anything but calm them—in fact, it made them anxious and stressed. The result was that on average, viewers smoked at least two cigarettes during the thirty-minute experiment. I was dumbstruck.

The interviews I had with them after the videos was a real education. What I learned was that everyone had already successfully gotten the message in life that smoking was bad for them. The video only repeated that message. Consider this: a smoking habit generally begins during the teenage years of rebellion and my trial participants were no different. The act of smoking is inextricably linked with the inner urge to rebel. This video, then, first pushed high anxiety buttons through the message that smoking is bad, then it also triggered the inherent response of a smoker's rebellion mindset: *turn against any information that pokes at my denial about what smoking is doing to me.* And so my viewers turned off the video and lit up the Marlboros.

What I learned then is what I know today: creating fear and guilt does not help people manage their bad habits. In fact, this only replicates dynamics that promoted their bad habits in the first place. Would you be helping a person with an alcohol problem by telling them how bad alcoholism is or how wicked or stupid they must be to have such a problem? No.

The video project's lesson has been confirmed through years I have spent helping people with addiction since then—the best ingredients of a positive wellness program are *offering hope* and *sharing skills*. What does work is to identify the problem they are struggling with as something that you understand and something that can be defeated. Then share with them the skills they can develop that can help that victory. Remind them that this achievable victory is not automatic through just acknowledgement; it requires action steps.

ADDICTION IN THE BRAIN AND BODY

The processes, cycles, and patterns that make up physical addiction are similar, no matter what the substance in question might be. Addictive substances quickly make their way to the pleasure centers of the brain, and once that relationship is established, so is the addiction. The area of the brain most interesting to note in this substance/brain relationship is called the *nucleus accumbens,* a part of the brain involved in the limbic system that is found in the lower back of the skull. If someone is in the habit of regular cigarette use, the impact of the nicotine on their nucleus accumbens is minor, not nearly as powerful as heroin's effect. But it is still strong enough for that person to start relying on cigarettes to shift their energy so they feel they can better deal with their physical and emotional needs.

The addictive substance doesn't affect just that part of the brain; the stimulation extends into other parts of the brain, including the *frontal lobe,* which is more domineering and controls organization and planning. When someone is addicted to smoking, it is their frontal lobe that does things like thinking about smoking even when they aren't smoking, planning for the next cigarette, and deciding when and how to purchase their next pack. If they are smoking secretively, the frontal lobe is also planning where to smoke and how to hide it. You can now well imagine how addiction to even more intense substances claims massive control of the frontal lobe, even to the point of a total obsession that devastates all other facets of life.

Smoking is like lighting multiple fires throughout the lungs and throat. These dozens of little fires expose internal organs, including heart and lungs, to the ashes and sparks. These little fires create burn-like blisters on tissues. In fact, those who are regularly exposed to fire—think, firefighters—can develop similar physical problems to smokers. Not surprisingly, our body does not like these smoky and ashy intruders. The immune system is alerted to these dangers. Then when these immune reactions create inflammatory battles, the body gets confused about what it is trying to fight off; the inflammation can aim at the very heart and lungs it was trying to protect in the first place. Thus smoking, or rather our body's reaction to smoking, can result in respiratory disease, heart disease, and cancer.

The recovery system that I have seen work best takes into account these complexities of the neural system and offers a plan based on brain dynamics. You see, we cannot rationally talk ourselves out of an addiction. Recovery requires retraining our brains and that takes two things: persistence and time. And as addiction often creates brain injury, big or small, and loss of motor coordination, a recovery system must also include treatment for inflammation and toxicity at those levels. This can look like practices to rehab our brains along with detoxing our bodies through nutrition and exercise. I want to share with you two cases to bring to life the addiction condition and a path out of it. First Lois, with an alcoholic addiction, and next Janet, with a nicotine addiction.

RESETTING FROM ALCOHOL

Lois had been drinking so often and for so long that she came to me with some severe behavioral control issues. Her willpower around alcohol was downright undetectable. Remember, her frontal lobe was completely hijacked by her addiction. She began her detox in an inpatient program, something that can be a wonderful place to start for those who relate to Lois. For some, similar success can also be achieved through an outpatient program—it all depends on the level of support that is needed. Once her program was complete, Lois continued to attend 12-Step meetings as often as she could. If she hadn't already been utilizing such a program, I would have included it in her reset wellness protocol for spiritual and social support.

I designed a wellness program for Lois aimed at strengthening the rhythmic elements in her brain. To break the looping behaviors of alcohol addiction was very important—a process she had begun in treatment—but the next step to bring her back into balance was to reset her behavioral patterns. Think of this as behaving *as if* you are a healthy person in order to become one! *What choice would a healthy person make right now?* you can ask yourself, or encourage those you are helping to ask themselves. Lois found positive music and intense drumming to have an amazing influence on her. There are often groups of drumming circles created for those in recovery. Other things that people I worked with have found helpful are vision quest experiences and sensory deprivation chambers.

REPLACING SMOKING PATTERNS

The process of nicotine recovery is slightly different than alcohol recovery because on the physical level, it is rarer that the nicotine itself is ingested (as alcohol is). To detox, Janet at first went through similar steps as Lois did. Both were urged to restructure their lives without the substance. I would never say that quitting smoking is easier than quitting alcohol. Like Lois, Janet had to detox her body and her social connections, and restructure her life around positive rhythmic patterns. Janet leaned heavily on exercise and nutrition. Exercise is important while trying to quit smoking, so I focused on three essential factors with her: breathing, exertion, and endurance. Lois used breathing exercises to de-stress, relax, and then mobilize in times of high demand. This helped her replace the use of nicotine to deal with stress with more empowering tools. This is a perfect example of the importance of offering skills to a person trying to recover from addiction. Exercise was also essential for Lois in order to strengthen her lungs from the damage smoking was causing them, and to repair her heart and cardiovascular system.

Recovery from nicotine addiction is based a great deal on why someone smokes in the first place. When helping yourself or someone else quit smoking, it is wise to investigate the *why* behind the habit. Typically, people smoke for five reasons.

1. *They fear the craving of the nicotine recovery*
   Craving inevitably comes with withdrawal, but you can give them hope with the reminder that it only lasts about seven days. Some skills you can share with them are the BAUD device, which is powerful in helping reset craving

loops in the brain. Relaxing breathing techniques can also help people get through this phase without undue frustration. Yes, there will likely be periods of anger outbursts and short fuses, but remind them, or yourself, that this phase can be managed and moved through.

2. *They use smoking to help with anxiety*

Relaxation practices that start to replace lighting up can be very helpful. Although it is an unhealthy version of these things, the act of smoking has its own cycles and rhythms—a cigarette with the sunrise, after every meal, and before bed. So help your patient or loved one find stimulating rhythmic activities that begin to replace the smoking habit: music, singing, dancing, breathing, or walking.

3. *They fear the boredom of not smoking*

Boredom relates to our environment. Maybe someone loved smoking on their back porch? Time to switch things up. Instead of smoking after dinner, they could take a walk around their neighborhood. Talking or humming to themselves, though perhaps not in public, can also help satisfy a bored attention span, as well as being healthy for the brain. Smoking support groups are also rich sources of ideas about how to manage boredom. In the end, the key is not only to cure boredom, but also to ignite purpose and passion. Encourage any recovering smoker to get involved with things they are passionate about or are interested in learning and discovering.

4. *They use smoking to help with depression*

In this case, more intensive movement exercises are wonderfully beneficial. The point is to stimulate the brain with rhythmic exercises that help break a sweat. Challenging physical movement gets the mind quickly focused on solutions rather than on sorrowful, past-focused thinking. The depressed ex-smoker might also find the *Peace and Joy* CD helpful, as well as positive music. Stay away from country western lyrics about lost love, long train rides, or beloved departed dogs, though!

5. *They want to be part of a social scene that includes other smokers*

Smokers can form a tight circle with its own ritualistic behaviors, such as taking smoke breaks together. Bumming a cigarette can be an easy way to make a connection at a party. But social smoking can keep a smoking habit going for years and create a mighty barrier to quitting. They must do the work of detaching from pleasing other smokers with their behavior. Someone might have to change friends or, at least, ask their friends for help. This task is not easy and must be acknowledged as such. Invite the recovering smoker to make new, non-smoking friends. Remind them that they can substitute cigarettes for a big glass of water, a nice walk, or some deep breathing inside during the social smoke breaks.

There *are* positive uses for nicotine, but not when it is delivered through smoking it. Research concludes that small amounts of nicotine found in natural substances are recognized and utilized by the body (George E. Barreto, 2015). In this form, nicotine has been shown to help the brain fog in Alzheimer's disease and other similar neurological cognitive problems.

I must add a warning about a supposedly helpful aid in stopping the smoking—vaping. Products made by Juul and other similar companies are as bad or worse for your health for similar reasons that smoking is bad. Similar to tobacco additives, vaping is full of dangerous chemicals. When introduced to the body through breathing, these chemicals offend the body and trigger an immune response just like smoking does—a response that can quickly go haywire and create major problems. In fact, I cannot recommend any inhalant approach as effective in stopping smoking, except one: take a straw that you might suck a drink through and breathe through it. You can even decorate it so it won't get lost!

ADDICTION RECOVERY WELLNESS STEPS

Stated in simple terms, the steps of addiction recovery from a wellness rhythms perspective are as follows. Give this list to those you are helping so they can remain focused on the things they *can* do, rather than just the things they cannot do.

1. Detoxify and strengthen your mind and body systems.

2. Deal positively with the craving process.

3. Identify the stressors and myths that brought you to this addiction and caused the loss of rhythmic energy in your life.

4. Identify the life choices that help you control the internal states of mind that your present life demands.

5. Create new rhythmic energies in your life every day.

6. Redefine your life, and possibly yourself!

7. Find friends and supporters who will help you get where you want to go.

I started this chapter with the story of making those "Stop Smoking" videos. The core shift I made then—and encourage you to make as you quit or help others do so—is that people with addictions are well-aware of the problems, so *act* is the verb to emphasize when giving guidance to them. I once had a coach who said, "Trying to argue with the referee, another member of our team, or the opposing team does not help us win a game. Just act like a football player and play the game!" I listened carefully because the lesson he was sharing is mission critical to those in recovery from addiction, or really anyone trying to get anything done. How did I write this book? I didn't talk about writing it, or think about writing it, or plan to write it, I just wrote it.

The thing about action is that it immediately prompts you to set goals, whether or not you realize it. The minute your foot hits the pavement, the questions arise: How far should I run? How hard should I run? How long should I run? These questions are living in the background and your answers to them cause you to adjust your energy output. If you have decided to run two miles in a short period, you will pace yourself differently than if you have decided to run two miles in an unlimited amount of time.

Similarly, sometimes people wonder how much time they should give themselves to stop smoking or drinking. The same questions arise about your goals with quitting as when you begin a run. If someone wants to take a year to stop smoking, then they must want to put out very little effort over a long period of time. If they want to stop tomorrow, then they must be ready to put out a huge amount of effort right away.

Recovery takes a lot of strength. Failure is not a reinforcing or inspiring experience; we all need to feel successful in order to be motivated to continue anything, especially recovery. Self-awareness is key in this process—being aware of our strength of energy, the effect of social pressures, and how much resilience we have to shift rhythms will all support moving out of addiction. Remind the person you are helping that if they feel weak when facing their addiction, they should focus on creating resolve before trying to quit a substance. If they feel strong and resourced, it is worth quitting tomorrow. If anxiety is diluting their empowerment, help them find some way of managing it (hopefully without introducing more medication into the situation). If someone needs permission socially to put down the cigarettes or the bottle, encourage them to find an ally or coach who will help empower them. Ending an addiction is a success you can truly define yourself by and take great power from. There is rhythmic bliss on the other side of dependency (G. Frank Lawlis, 2015).

CHAPTER 12

EXPLORE SELF-DISCOVERY

I have been and still am a seeker, but I have ceased to question stars and books; I have begun to listen to the teaching my blood whispers to me.
–Hermann Hesse, *Demian*

In my research on body and brain rhythms, I've come to realize that there is no greater transformative power than self-knowledge. Our lives include successes and failures, risks and mistakes, growth opportunities and setbacks, as well as challenges to overcome. In these conditions, balance is the ability to respond according to our true goals and passions. This is driven by an endless process of self-discovery.

To remain without this self-knowledge can lead to an unfulfilled, depressing, and ultimately, lonely life, in which we simply go through the motions of the everyday with no sense of adventure or discovery. Underlying any societally defined success we may have achieved, each person has a story to tell. The part of the American Dream that I like to emphasize is our ability to overcome challenges by staying true to our vision and navigating by that star. Whether you're helping yourself, your loved ones, or your patients, true wellness comes from identifying and attaining the goals that arise from within. This requires a connection to who we are.

RESILIENCE IS WHAT MAKES DREAMS COME TRUE

Growing up, Joe and his family didn't have much, but theirs was a deeply spiritual household where hard work and family love were sacred. Although Joe, like many of his peers, had his flirtations with alcohol, drugs, and other questionable decision-making, on the whole he was a fellow who made sound choices and seemed destined for a modest yet stable and satisfying life. But Joe wanted something more. He had a powerful self-concept and believed in his future.

From his first job as a paperboy, he took his work seriously and built on his early successes. His family believed in education, so Joe went to college and earned an undergraduate degree while working full-time. By the age of twenty, he had earned a contractor's license and made a name, as well as a comfortable life, for himself. After a tornado laid his town flat, he led its reconstruction and achieved a status as a local hero.

Having come from a strong family background, it was just a matter of time before Joe got married. But it didn't last. His new wife didn't recognize Joe's true passions or goals—perhaps because Joe didn't quite recognize them himself. His business leveled out and he continued on in construction, respected and financially stable. And yet he felt tugged by a sense of wanting more…he just wasn't sure what that was.

Joe struggled with his sense of purpose. But what was next? His business had expanded to neighboring towns and then throughout the county. This helped him realize how satisfying being in business can be when offering reliable services that delight customers. As his interest shifted from construction to business, he began entertaining the idea of obtaining an MBA and taking the effort to a national level. He had fallen in love with another woman, the "right one" this time, but should he burden his new marriage with student debt by going back to school for a graduate degree? His family certainly was in no financial position to help. And besides, despite his experience, could a hammer-and-nails guy like Joe even handle the rigors of business school? For the first time in his life, Joe felt lost, torn between dreams and doubt. And there was no one who could tell him what he ought to do.

Joe is not the first nor the last person to come up against such an obstacle. Even Moses, adopted as a young child, raised in a king's house, revered for his intelligence and accomplishments, and destined for the throne himself, struggled to find a sense of belonging. He felt more of a kinship with the enslaved Hebrews than with the royal family into which he had been adopted. It was only after his exile in the desert that Moses was able to learn his true purpose: to lead those slaves, his people, out of Egypt and to the promised land. It is said that Moses was given his purpose by God. Not all journeys of self-discovery are directly inspired by the divine, but we all must endeavor to take them just the same.

Joe took a long time to realize that he too was born to be a leader. But, eventually, he did go back to school. He earned a graduate degree and succeeded beyond his wildest dreams. But much more than the material success, fame, and influence he now holds around the world, it is his ability to *lead others into their own power* that brings Joe his greatest reward. Like Joe, as we navigate our own journeys and achieve some success, we then realize the value of helping and guiding others on their paths.

DOORS OF SELF-DISCOVERY

There are a number of useful tools and practices to help us walk through the threshold of our innermost motivations. In my fifty years as a psychologist, I've seen countless people like Joe use personality tests and other assessments to quantify and reveal their strengths, true goals, and passions. I'd like to offer a simple and fun exercise called the Color Test for Self-Discovery, which offers a glimpse of our self-concept. Try the test for yourself and offer it to family members and patients.

Instructions
Using the grid below, you'll be comparing eight colors: Black (BL), Light Blue (LB). Dark Blue (DB), Brown (BR), Red (R), Light Green (LG), Dark Green (DG), and White (W). The colors are arranged horizontally and vertically, like a multiplication table. At each point where two colors intersect, write in the initials for the one you prefer. (I've X'd out the boxes where a color meets itself.) After filling in the boxes, total the number of times the color at the top of each column appears again in that column, and write that total below that column.

	BL	LB	DB	BR	R	LG	DG	W
BL	XX							
LB		XX						
DB			XX					
BR				XX				
R					XX			
LG						XX		
DG							XX	
W								XX
Total								

Here's a sample filled out by a friend of mine, Natalie. In her comparisons, she chose White more than any other color.

	BL	LB	DB	BR	R	LG	DG	W
BL	XX	LB	DB	BR	R	LG	DG	W
LB	LB	XX	LB	LB	R	LB	LB	W
DB	DB	LB	XX	DB	DB	DB	DB	W
BR	BR	LB	DB	XX	BR	LG	DG	W
R	R	R	DB	BR	XX	LG	DG	R
LG	LG	LB	DB	LG	LG	XX	DG	W
DG	DG	LB	DB	DG	DG	DG	XX	W
W	W	W	W	W	R	W	W	XX
Total	BL x 0	LB x 5	DB x5	BR x 2	R x 3	LG x 3	DG x 2	W x 6

Natalie's choice signifies that she needs purity of thought to make decisions. She wants to get as much information about a situation or person as possible, sometimes extensively, to the point of ruminating about her choices. As a leader, she takes great pains to try and incorporate other people's ideas and thoughts. In general, she is an optimistic person who feels gratitude for life and values her friends tremendously.

Interpretations

Try this test for yourself and, if you find it helpful, ask others to do so also. Here are the basic interpretations, which are brief but have profound ways of showing up in our lives. To further your understanding of them, you might contemplate the expansive effects of these styles and see if you can witness them in action.

> **Black** choices indicate that a person may tend to see the world as a mysterious place. On the one hand, they could be cautious and skeptical, but on the other, they might relish the mystery of the unknown.

> **Light Blue** is the color of the sky and of shallow water, and people who choose it may tend to want complete transparency in relationships or business. They value trust and openness.

> **Dark Blue**, the color of deeper water, indicates a person who prefers to explore others in depth, even if it takes a while. People who choose Dark Blue also deepen their understanding of issues and situations as things change.

> **Brown** is the color of earth. Those who choose it have simple needs and find pleasure in sincere relationships. (Think "salt of the earth.") They tend to be nurturing and forgiving, and able to put aside their own needs.

Red is the color of blood and passion. A person who favors red is a risk taker who lives "on the edge," or "in the moment." Their quick smile or a flash of their eyes makes them charming, even when their lust for life may be ill-timed.

Light Green indicates that a person loves new life, in nature, work, and relationships. The excitement of a new project may lead them to entrepreneurship, although they may move on once the excitement wears off. The same might be true in friendships or romance.

Dark Green is the color of the harvest, indicating an affinity for more mature people and for well-established businesses or ongoing projects. Dark Green folks are organized, and they value loyalty, teamwork, and long-term relationships.

White is the combination of all other colors into light. People who favor white tend to seek out spiritual answers and see a higher dimension or purpose to their work and lives. They invest themselves fully into all aspects of their own and others' lives through creativity, love, and support.

These colors indicate what inspires, motivates, and propels us. Knowing more about what engages our passions can help us stay aware of our inner truth as we make life decisions and even interact with each other on a daily basis. It's important to ask ourselves and others, "What really gets you going?" This is how we can harness our natural fuel and travel in the direction of our dreams. But while identifying those dreams and accessing the resources we need to reach them is an inner process, it still requires some assistance.

SOLITUDE AND VISION QUESTS

Moses received his wake-up call and purpose straight from God. The rest of us must also search for ways to receive information *transpersonally*—that is, from beyond our conscious selves. The key to full self-discovery is in our ability to receive this sort of guidance.

One of the ways we open the door to discovery for ourselves and others is through solitude. Anyone who's ever felt that they "just want to be alone for a while" has recognized that there is peace—and likely, clarity—to be had in stepping away for a time. There are many self-discovery programs that take inspiration from traditional rites of passage, in which a young person sets out to find his or her purpose in life. Often these programs center around a wilderness experience of three days or more. The solo traveler carries little beyond basic survival gear, sometimes even just a canteen of water. And although traditions of killing bears or other wild animals are long gone, the experience is intense and fraught with real and potentially dangerous challenges.

Out of respect for tribal traditions, I won't discuss particular rituals and symbols in detail, but there is one modern ritual that is astoundingly transformative and powerful. The late anthropologist Michael Harner, who brought shamanism into contemporary healing, took participants on their journeys not through physical challenges in foreign environments, but deep within their subconscious minds. I encourage you to try this, and then offer it to loved ones and patients.

Offer instructions ahead of time to the person going on the quest so that nothing is said during the ritual. The leader or practitioner remains with the person and may drum rhythmically to enhance the imagery of the journey. There may be others present and drumming as well, but even in this group setting, the journey itself will be a completely solitary experience.

Instructions for Inner Journeying

Lie down with your eyes closed. Then with your imagination, seek out and find a hole in the ground, such as a cave, an animal burrow, or a crack between rocks. You may be tempted to investigate, but you must enter the opening and continue along without stopping.

After a while, you will emerge at another place on Earth. Explore your new surroundings. If an animal appears, ask if it will be your spirit ally. If it declines, wait for another animal to come. Eventually, one will agree to be your ally. You may ask the animal for guidance about your mission, or about anything you choose. The animal may take you on a revealing adventure or guide you to another creature or being who has something to tell you.

A special drum beat will signal that it's time to come back. Thank the animal, then re-enter the hole and make your way back to the place you started. When you feel that you are back, open your eyes.

After the journey, discuss the animal and the interaction with it. The person who has undergone the journey and identified their spirit ally should research traits of that animal and how it lives. Sometimes the qualities and attributes revealed about oneself are surprising, enlightening, and empowering.

SENSORY DEPRIVATION EXPERIENCE

Sensory deprivation also provides the solitude needed, not through an interactive journey, but through the deliberate removal of external stimuli. Listening to *Entropy* (www.mind-bodybylawlis.com) is an ideal way to augment the deprivation environment, as it helps the listener reach that deep, almost unconscious state, like sleep, in which the mind can grasp information from within. For an hour or more, simply relax and listen for words of wisdom to arise.

THE ONGOING PROCESS OF SELF DISCOVERY

Self-discovery is not a moment in time, a single *Aha!* moment in which every last mystery is solved, every detail revealed. It is a process over the course of a lifetime, because we change. Our bodies, our brains, our relationships, and our world are all in a constant state of change. The only thing that never changes is the fact that nothing stays the same.

So be careful not to get trapped in a fixed mindset about yourself, or about anyone or anything. If you do, you might miss out on any number of amazing opportunities and experiences. If you start a career and, a few years later, realize it's not what you expected—or that what you want has fundamentally changed—does it really makes sense to stay in it? The psychologist Abraham Maslow wrote about the hierarchy of needs, with one of his central tenets being that our needs change as we change.

It may seem like some of our social structures keep you, your loved ones, or your patients from exploring and finding a true self. And that's why some solitude is so crucial to have in your life. Without it, how do we know what is right—*for us?*

Searching for purpose, self-concept, and true happiness— not someone else's definition of it—can be a daunting prospect, but it's also thrilling and so rewarding. Each season of life brings new beginnings and new passions. Each is a new chance to live in the beat of life, and in the rhythms of the universe that exist around us and live through us.

CHAPTER 13

CULTIVATE RELATIONSHIPS

Your task is not to seek for love, but merely to seek and find
all the barriers within yourself that you have built against it.
—Rumi

Love is a powerful source of healing. Love appears to have its own energies, sourced from our spirit and moving through our heart and body, inspiring us to rise above stress, petty concerns, and sometimes, even disease. No research is needed for us to know this, though the studies do verify the irreplaceable power of love in the healing process. Research finds that survival rates when we are impacted by illness and trauma are increased with the presence of stable and supportive relationships (Cloitre, 2008). Love and our need for it is as mysterious as it is perceivable. It impacts every aspect of our lives, including our physical and psychological well-being.

Relationships between human beings have transpersonal rhythms to them, which may be invisible but are essentially tied to wellness outcomes. Sometimes the rhythmic powers of a relationship are easy to increase because of the structure of the relationship itself. Dancing is an example. As a teenager I thought of myself as a good dancer, but when I got to college, there was a new dance called the North Texas Push. I tried as hard as I could, but never understood the steps. As I stumbled on the feet of my date, I felt the relationship suffering. On the other hand, when in later years, I knew the steps and rules in ballroom dancing, several relationships blossomed from those encounters. Another rhythm that effects relationship is the rhythm of music. Some of the most emotive music of all time follows the pace of the heartbeat. Love affairs often grow out of shared musical experiences, like singing together. Relationship rhythms are also nurtured by experiencing natural rhythms together: watching the moon and stars moving through the night sky, or strolling together down a scenic path. Or in the case of business relationships, we can rhythmically work together to complete multifaceted projects on time.

RHYTHMS OF BUSINESS RELATIONSHIPS

Business relationships can be understood and made to work well, but the dynamics are complex. These interactions are based on a hierarchy of power; if one knows the rules of that hierarchy, the relationship can be very productive. There are three leadership styles which your boss or supervisor, or you, if you are the boss, embodies: authoritative, democratic, and permissive. Ideally, a leader is a happy balance of these energies, but more typically, a leader is predominantly one type. If someone you are helping reset wellness rhythms is having challenges at work, encourage them to first analyze which types are at play around them in the workplace, or which type they are themselves.

The authoritative style of supervision is one in which the supervisor holds all the power and responsibility for success within himself or herself. This style is common in the military and works well there, as this style is in tune with the military system as a whole. If the subordinate wants a relationship to work most rhythmically, they must follow the rules and adhere to this principle. They must serve without expectation of perhaps ever sharing the responsibilities or power. They must do the supervisor's directives to the best of their ability.

The democratic supervisor, on the other hand, shares the responsibilities and power of the demands on the relationship. For example, if something is off between someone and their democratic boss, the boss might bring it up or they might wait and let the employee bring it up—they expect the tasks and the emotional labor of the job to be shared. This relationship functions similar to how a team operates. In order for the relationship to be rhythmic, a subordinate to this leadership style must participate in the responsibilities and power. The supervisor will expect them to speak up with their ideas and share some success or failure. The more responsibility taken by the employee, the better the relationship will evolve. This relationship is typically most productive business-wise, but it is less personal because the focus of the relationship is usually on the goals, not on mentorship.

The permissive leader rests all the responsibilities of the relationship on the subordinate, blaming failure or success on them. The most rhythmic condition of this dynamic demands that the employee be willing to undertake the mission of the relationship as their own and not expect support from above. This position can be fruitful if someone wants power and freedom to do things in their own way; it can be frustrating and lonely if they expect or need direction.

Consider that these leadership types suggest subordinate types as well: the submissive, the team player, and the self-starter. The dynamics between these types of leading and working can be positive and embraced. However, the rhythmic energy becomes negative when the rules of the structure are not met. For example, if a team player has an authoritative leader, there will be friction. If a submissive person has a democratic leader, they are likely to feel a vacuum of energy in the relationship (Sweney, 1970).

I have described these three leadership archetypes as if they were personality types, but ideally, all three energies are combined and present in any one person, creating a blend of abilities that can be used while leading a wide range of employees. Such a well-rounded individual would have the skills to tap into the power of the relationship rhythm, regardless of the subordinate present.

RHYTHMS OF LOVE RELATIONSHIPS

When I say "love relationships" I mean committed couples who feel they are in love with each other and are nurturing a relationship, based on love, that they wish to grow. I believe that love relationships have the power to grow in intensity and magnitude, which is the hope and desire of the partners involved, but of course, the rules are harder to learn. It is not as simple as figuring out a partner's leadership style and asking the other partner to bend to that. Love relationship rhythms are complicated because they involve personal desire and preference, as well as the culture and family pattern of each individual partner.

To bring to life the skills and theories of love relationships, I have brought the wisdom and insight of Joyce Buckner into this chapter (Buckner, 2004). Dr. Buckner has been a practicing psychologist for marriage counseling for thirty-five years, and has amazing perspective on how people can nurture their love rhythms over years.

I became involved in the field of marriage counseling during the era in which researchers became interested in the all-important question, *What makes marriages work and fail?* I was intrigued by the earth-shattering statistic that emerged at the time. For the first time in United States history, 50 percent of marriages, the researchers said, were ending in divorce. At the time, I was an associate professor of psychology at Texas Tech University and was supervising graduate students who were looking for topics to study. Many them were as interested in the recent divorce statistics as I was, so we decided to drill into the essence of married life and speak to couples who had been married for more than fifty years about their experience of keeping their love alive. Although it was Texas, and each couples' answers were primarily influenced by their agrarian lifestyle, there was much to be learned from their histories.

A main pattern we noticed in our research was the magic of support in long-lasting love—one of the principles of committed relationships was the assumption that each of the partners dedicated themselves to the support of the other. Again and again, these principles came to life in the stories of the people we spoke to. One of the basic questions we asked in the interviews was for a description of the couples' daily life. In one of our first interviews, the wife began describing a typical morning for them before they had retired.

"We got started about 4:00 a.m. because we had to milk the cows. Then we got breakfast, which was oatmeal."

I broke in and asked why she said *oatmeal*, specifically.

"Because we always had oatmeal," she replied.

To which her husband said, "Yeah, we always had oatmeal, although I got tired of it."

The wife became shocked. "Why in hell didn't you tell me? This is the first time you said that in fifty years!"

"Well, you seemed to like making it, and I figured I could be flexible. After all, you were doing it for me, so why should I complain? I didn't want you to feel bad."

His first remark—"I figured I could be flexible"—demonstrated his commitment to being happy, no matter what he ate for breakfast. And the rest—"you were doing it for me" and "I didn't want you to feel bad"—demonstrated his gratitude for his wife's actions and his support of her.

The theme of having concern for one's partner was evident throughout our research. It is the root of this chapter. If we value our love relationships, we should nurture them in heart, mind, and soul everyday of our lives.

RULES OF LOVE GROWTH

Romantic love rhythms emerge in two stages: the formation of a love rhythm—falling in love—and learning how to nurture that love rhythm—keeping yourself in love. During the first stage, the love rhythm seems to be creating itself, perhaps as if by magic. Although it is not a very romantic analysis, the love is probably not happening magically, but through unconscious selections the lovers are making based on their own history. My studies have led me to some interesting conclusions about the nature of partner selection, including body smells, hair color, resemblance to or difference from parents, and complementary or similar scores on personality tests. Specific situations in which people are interacting about common interests, such as political or religious concerns, also draw people together.

During my tenure at Texas Tech, I created a questionnaire called The Four Relationships Test. Once taken, the questionnaire would determine at what stage the answerer's love relationship was. There were four dimensions to the quiz: prestige/respect, identification, sexual/affectionate, and problem-solving. Although this quiz is now out of print, the principles it brought to life are still full of relational rhythm wisdom.

- Prestige/respect rhythms exist in relationships in which there is a lot of respect for each other's wisdom, prestige, and power energies.

- The identification aspect is rhythmically present when the partners have kinship to the energy of a common cause.

- The sexual/affectionate rhythm involves caring and nurturing.

- The problem-solving rhythm includes interactions in which creative solutions are shared through mutual energies.

During the end of stage one of relationships, when the rhythm that was seeming to beat on its own accord is just starting to slow down, the quiz revealed one of two things: either the relationship had only one of the four rhythms going for it and would fade away, or there was more than one rhythm present and, if this was the case, the relationship would survive and enter stage two. You see, stage one of love rhythms has no set rules or time-stamp; it generates itself and survives as long as the purpose driving it survives. It can last as long as sexual energies live on (which is sometimes only ten minutes!) if that is the inspiration for its creation. Or it can last years if the rhythm it is tapped into is motivating enough for the two people involved. For instance, if both partners are utterly motivated by the prestige/respect rhythm and both find that having each other as allies at networking events and speaking conferences, then their stage one relationship could last a lifetime—but only if both are satisfied with that being their only rhythmic connection.

Stage two is the growth stage of love relationship rhythms and does have set rules about what benefits or hinders that growth. The following rules, which I call the *do not* rules, hinder relational rhythm growth.

- ◆ ***Do not* criticize the other person.** Criticism, regardless of intention, diminishes the energy of love relationships. The main healing power of the love rhythm is the opposite of criticism; it is support. Relational energy, as well as self-esteem, is lost through criticism. While it may have been fashionable in the '70s to "fully express opinion," in a relationship, such thoughtlessness indicates self-absorption and the valuing of self-expression over care for another.

- ◆ ***Do not* disappear.** If someone was neglected in childhood, they tend to shut off their feelings and emotions when someone close to them is directing discomfort toward them. If someone was left alone too much as a child, they may have had to become unnaturally strong and stoic in order to survive. This may have empowered them personally, but may mean they tend to escape emotionally when intensity arises. But in escaping, they are essentially abandoning their partner because they are not able to respond or produce empathy. This will only cause the upset partner to amplify their feelings in order to be heard. A kind of emotional vacuum appears between the distancer and the expresser and the rhythm is stalled.

- ◆ ***Do not* rush to conclusions.** Problem-solving's number one enemy is jumping to conclusions.

When one or both people in a love relationship do not feel that their feelings or positions are understood, an impasse forms. We can become so defensive that we anticipate being challenged, rather than seeking to understand. We may feel that our honor, or even our survival, is being challenged. Such a situation creates a blockage of rhythms. In order for the partners to proceed, the stagnation must be cleared out.

RHYTHMS OF PROMISE IN RELATIONSHIP

Energy rhythms flow naturally between people, but they are sensitive things and need nurturing and direction. I would like to share with you tools and approaches that are nurturing for relationship rhythms, practices that can help you or a patient you are helping corral the energy dynamics toward growth and positivity.

Relax Your Environment and Yourself

Encourage those you are helping to create around themselves a relaxed environment for positive rhythms. For example, I enjoy the influence of soft music, especially songs by my wife and people I have positive histories with. Music that we love stimulates positive memories in our limbic systems and helps us focus on growth. The colors around us also influence our rhythms—think of wall color and décor. As seen in Native American culture and in the nature all around us, green is connected with a state of growth. Some research has shown that blue stimulates the brain-waking frequencies. Perhaps the depression that affects so many and can be such a major cause of stress in relationships would be soothed by more blue in one's space.

Another important element of our environments are the other life forms we live with—plants (real ones are always best) and animals. It has been found that plants react to the emotions of the humans around them and exude subtly different scents as their contribution to balance their environments. And there is nothing so comforting as petting the furry coat or hide of a beloved animal. Skin-on-skin contact takes us back to the motherly caress, going beyond what our cognitive processes can comprehend.

If a couple seeks out relationship counseling, it means they are probably feeling a lot of stress in the relationship. Being in counseling can even add to the stress at first. In order to bring down those levels, I sometimes hook both partners up to a biofeedback device that measures stress levels. My device of choice measures finger temperature, which I find is easiest and least expensive for the couples.

How does it work? Temperature is related to blood vessel dilation. When a person experiences stress, these vessels constrict and the hand typically becomes colder. The procedure is to wrap the ring finger with the temperature monitor bud and read the numbers attached to the monitor. Do this for both members of the couple. The sure-proof reading for stress is any reading that comes in under 90 degrees Fahrenheit. Then, in the counseling session, if the temperature dips below 90 degrees, I pause the conversation. No one is allowed to react to anything said, and they must focus on relaxing and allowing the temperature to rise again before we can resume. Sometimes people come in already reading below 90 degrees, and I lead a short destressing process before we begin, such as deep breathing. It is interesting to note that lying is stressful and may cause a temperature dip as well! The power of keeping themselves in a relaxed rhythm during a session gives the participants an amazing chance to speak more mindfully and think more clearly and creatively about each other.

Communicate Rhythmically

The unfolding process of learning to understanding oneself and another *is* the richness of relationship. Exchanging empathic communication in a flowing, rhythmic nature is a dance. When we take turns with our partner to define and describe events and the emotions they brought up, we learn about ourselves, we learn about them, and we learn about the underlying assumptions and myths at play in our particular partnership. Ideally, this rhythm looks like this: One person explains some event or aspect of the relationship, usually communicating some pain or confusion along with it. The other person clarifies by noting the emotion expressed and verifying the other's pain. The first person either validates the response or restates the concern in an effort to be better understood. The ritual continues until there is a mutual agreement. Here are two ways it can go:

> *Person 1: "I don't know why you flirt with women when we are socializing. It hurts and is embarrassing."*

> *Person 2: "I think you are telling me that when I don't give you my full attention when we're out, you feel like I'm ignoring you and like I prefer others. Is that right?"*

Person 1: "Well, no and yes. I feel that you are doing it to hurt me and show me that you can find someone else better. Does that make sense?"

Person 2: "I am so sorry if that was how you felt because I thought I was pleasing you by being so friendly. When we were dating, you told me you liked how friendly I was. I want you to be proud of me and you know how shy I am. I guess I was overdoing it."

Person 1: "I think you understand me better."

Person 2: "Let's think of some way you can feel safer. I want to feel like your champion."

Another example:

Person 1: "When we go out, you always make a big deal of what I'm wearing, how my hair is combed, if my shoes are polished. I feel smothered with your attention to how I look. It makes me feel like I'm incompetent to take care of myself."

Person 2: "What I hear is you telling yourself that you don't care how people see you."

Person 1: "Absolutely not. I do care, but I feel that my self-esteem goes down the toilet when you tell me how I should be seen."

Person 2: "OK, I get it. You want me to just not care."

Person 1: "No, I want you to care, but not take responsibility. It's my job to look good. You can be my consultant. I value your view, but I am responsible."

Person 2: "Oh, I can do that."

Notice how the listener (Person 2 in both cases) focused on really understanding what Person 1 was bringing to them. Person 1 focused on articulating what they *really* meant. The back-and-forth had a higher goal in mind—circling around clarity and insight, rather than spiraling into unhelpful jabs and side comments.

Bring Warmth and Feed the Senses

Intensifying and nurturing relational rhythms does not just happen through words, though it often still happens through the voice. For me, the low register of how the Spanish language is used to express love conveys a soothing, sexy, caring intention. When I taught counseling skills, I often suggested to students that they get speaking lessons from the theatre department, especially from women. Anxiety is telegraphed through high, squeaky, and speedy vocal rhythms. I will never forget one student who demonstrated his hypnosis procedure, for which he was very proud, but he sounded like an auctioneer or racing commentator. When speaking with a partner, taking a breath or two communicates caring better than using all the words in the dictionary. How we speak is perhaps as important as what we say.

Apart from the voice, care is shown by looking into a person's eyes, as if desiring to see the other's heart. Leaning towards another, appropriately, shows intentional focus on what they are feeling and saying. If permission has be given, touching a person on his or her hand or arm can be extremely powerful. My research shows that the pheromone, or body scent, of a relaxed person is more powerful and magnetizing than that of a sexually aroused or anxious person. The pheromones of the relaxed are appealing and unconsciously register as more caring to those around them. I don't know if there is a perfume that offers such a message; if there is, I would invest in it.

Be Authentic and Transcend

Authenticity, shared without opinion or condition, is a major stimulus to relationship rhythms. Authenticity is not an opinion that holds any value or harm for anyone else or a statement that it is applicable to anyone else's life. Sometimes we get authenticity confused with honesty. Authenticity does require honesty with oneself, but it also requires an impulse to share responsibly thoughts that are supportive of the rhythm of the relationship. For example, being authentic does not mean sharing one's view of the Civil War or what one's grandfather thought about the Civil War; it is sharing a thought or feeling that might convey some insight that has emerged from oneself. See if you can hear it here:

- "As you were explaining your thoughts, I had a deep sense of pain for you because of how I would feel if my mother had told me that when I was as young."

- "When I picture having the dream you had, I might interpret this figure as being fearful because you were running away from it. What do you think?"

♦ "I don't know what you should do, but I would hope for you that you could give up some anger and forgive what is past so you can look forward to the future."

This last example brings me to my final piece of advice about nurturing healthy relationship rhythms. *Transcending* means to rise above the chaos and feelings of the past so we can see the future. Remind yourself and encourage those you are working with to support to forgive the offenses they have endured in their relationships and create a new history. As Dr. Phil McGraw famously asks the guests on his show, "Do you want to be right, or do you want to be happy?" In this spirit, we demonstrate to our partner that we see the relationship as a priority in our life and are willing to nurture it above all else.

THE CIRCLE OF LOVE

Love rhythms evolve through life and its many challenges. There is a time when relationships come and go. This is a time for independence, when we are the self-sufficient hero of our own journeys. There are also times when relationships call on us for caring and nurturance, such as during illness. We may then discover in ourselves new energy for caring. I remember caring for my late wife, Lorri, and the tremendous demands it made on me. I had to extend every ounce of energy for the care of her brain disease, without the need for anything in return. I was grateful for the nurturing and caring rhythm it elicited in me. Now I am in the casualty stage; I am the one asking for help from my beloved wife, Susan, and deepening my love rhythms each day.

The circling rhythms of relationship often occur several times a day. The rhythm of the daily give and take, grounded in the power of love, is intensely healing. The healing work of a shared past can become part of present insight and, by growing gratitude for each other, we can relate in an evolving way with great joy.

CONCLUSION

All challenges in our lives can help us grow into wisdom. By embracing the constancy of change, and even learning how it is a force for healing, we can stave off the greatest source of disharmony and illness. While the issues I described in this book might currently disrupt everything, we have the natural resources to work with them. If that wasn't the case, humankind would have become extinct long ago.

Whenever we need help, for any life challenge, we are experiencing a knot in the thread of health that runs through our beings. If that knot tightens, or gets bigger, through the momentum of imbalanced practices in life, our health will continue toward negative results. This is when we can intervene—but not only to resolve the challenge. We can also integrate its essential changes to step toward a life of greater balance and insight.

This is the educational aspect of human development, which continues throughout our lives. We face many unique challenges along the way, yet the earth-rhythm tools for growing in harmony within ourselves are common to all. The issues we face have histories that go back to the beginning of recorded history, and so do the world wisdom approaches to healing them. Most important, these healing methods resolved the causes of imbalance and illness instead of their symptoms. The healing process has been around as long as we have, and cultures that worked with them—instead of forcing them or substituting them—offered healing as a powerful pathway to wisdom.

While the world was vastly simpler even a few decades ago, much less two millennia ago, diseases and trauma still threatened the lives of our predecessors and ancestors. Today, we have more techniques, but diseases and trauma still rage on as evolving germs and tragically demanding lifestyles require more than the expensive potions we buy at the local drugstore can solve. Each body-mind system is more than a group of single cells. Complexes of systems form life *together,* serving each other and the greater purpose of wellness. We have been focusing disease research on strictly cellular levels, which is like studying sparkplugs to solve traffic jams. We need a revolution in the way we view, treat, and experience illness and health.

THE CASE FOR A WELLNESS REVOLUTION

We are still babes in the woods when we try to define health and determine what is good for us and what is not. Our medical system has told us that we can't be sad or we are sick. We also cannot be happy all the time or else we are sicker. We must poop every day or we are sick, and we can't poop more or we are sick with something else.

Our measurements for wellness are still extremely primitive for this day and age. The thermometer measures the heat in our bodies, which is hardly translatable to diagnosing specific diseases, so we take our children to doctors who insist on some antibiotic to cure the heat. But after one round of antibiotics, negative effects on gut health can persist for years in children and sometimes in adults.

We still use the pressure cuff, which is unreliable for a daily measure and offers no cause or treatment indication when it reads high or low, as both are bad and caused by completely different reasons. There needs to be something better to cure blood pressure issues, like investigating the cause. Sometimes high blood pressure has to do with a systematic inflammatory issue and sometimes it's an emotional response to stress events, but our current medicines don't account for causes, which makes them more dangerous to the rest of the body.

Some years ago, there was controversy in medicine over two ways to focus attention for healing humans: attacking the disease (germ) or strengthening the host's defense (body) against the invader. Before I create a new controversy, I have to say that this is not a contest nor an election. My life has been saved by both camps, and I have great gratitude for their services and training. I chose a personal physician who applies the strategy of strengthening my mind and body against the blows of disease invaders. But American medical schools most often take an attacking approach, as it is probably more lucrative in the long run because of the huge research base required and the prestige factor. The American medical community focuses on getting rid of any invader (with the exception of vaccines, which are a defense) and Eastern medicine chooses to strengthen the body, so it overcomes attacks with its own healing ability.

These two sides of medicinal focus have been generally divided as "acute" and "chronic" medical care. Acute medical care addresses the issues that need urgent care and curative results in a short period of time, such as heart attacks, broken limbs, poisoning, and strokes. This is the stuff of movies and television because there is no need to see the hard times of rehabilitation. The healer is the hero, and he gets the girl, so to speak.

Chronic disease medicine usually targets long-term effects from lifestyle changes and recovery approaches. It might take years to resolve some types of illness or injury and often at some expense, as with brain injury, loss of limbs, war trauma, addictions, type 2 diabetes, and obesity. The patient does not emerge completely whole, but with limitations. I have sadly observed that patients in these difficult human experiences receive much of the blame for their condition, though they ought to be raised to the status of a hero, since they deserve credit for any healing success. Patients therefore dismiss how healing it can be to accept that we need to function in a new way that is optimal for our changed condition.

I must mention that medical care is also important for patients whose healing effort is not to recover from disease, but to go through the process of dying. This "palliative" care can offer immense benefit, whether through reduced pain and stress or feelings of resolution and spiritual connection, when it has a peaceful passage as its goal. Death comes to us all, and there is no need to view its inevitable arrival as an enemy to forever attack at all cost to quality of life.

The controversy over vaccines illustrates the tension in modern medicine, as parents and the medical profession argue about who knows best when it comes to a child's health. I mention this issue because it goes to the heart of the philosophy of medical care and the possible role of the wellness approach for national well-being. While, as in all things, I advocate balance, we must acknowledge that, when we use medicine to protect the body from a disease, we are making the decision that the body needs help defending itself, therefore weakening the natural system. Until the vaccines were invented, children were expected to have the childhood diseases (measles, mumps, chicken pox, and so on) with the expectation that they would strengthen their immune systems by developing white blood cell (WBC) count code and never have them again. If we are attacked by a disease or something else and we fight it, we are strengthened. However, if we lose, we may be weaker and even die. The choice in preventative care comes down to the severity of the disease and the health of our bodies to resist.

I find that treatment success is more based on how strong we are and only secondarily on the method. If the basic wellness factor is lifestyle, we have the potential for control. There is defensive action we can take against addiction, chronic pain, obesity, some cancer categories, diabetes, quality of life, and others. Taking advantage of our wellness resources can help our nation more effectively manage disease in both acute and chronic situations, perhaps in palliative care as well.

Authority for recommending medical interventions in consumer health care has been designated to the Food and Drug Administration (FDA) and, unfortunately, their process calls solely for the "Golden Standard" method of proving an effective treatment. The high cost of entry to meet requirements bars programs that don't have a profit motive involved. We can see the glaring error in this approach in the opioid epidemic, as well as the mass inefficiency of the whole system's bias against natural components.

The biggest flaw in this arrangement is the insistence on the single-drug approach applied in elementary statistics. It would be more efficient to use multiple variant statistics in their strategies, and studies that look at multiple cross-organ effects, as well as long-term effects and side effects. We generally have no clue what happens in children who are treated with adult drugs before their brains have matured. We also all understand that drug effects impact more than one system. For example, anti-depressive drugs usually cause weight gain and, for some groups like patients with PTSD, actually induce suicidal thought behaviors and harm cognitive performance. Some statin drugs produce cognitive decline and anxiety. Yet we choose to warn patients in small print and ask them to live with effects, rather than arrive at understandings for why they happen and how we might create better treatments that don't compromise another aspect of wellness.

Our medical system could better recognize the downfall of our use of parametric statistics that requires so many subjects to reach significance (false negatives results) or virtually guarantee positive results (false positive results). There have been many articles that show methodologies of one subject over time can indicate evidence for consideration.

We have models that show wellness approaches work to boost economic health. The model I worked toward in Japan strengthened its economy, as it countered the effects of stress on workers' bodies. Wellness approaches in US industries show a positive impact on efficiency through profits. This too must be taken into account when assessing a nation's approach to health care.

THE OUTCOMES OF A FUNDAMENTAL SHIFT ARE ENDLESS

I am known as an experimenter of methods for recovery in many types of cases, and have been curious enough to attempt a variety of approaches that are outside traditional American methods. These are not contradictory to traditional health care; they add approaches to enhance outcomes. Many of these have outstanding results, but don't receive formal attention from entities like the FDA, even if they might be considered breakthroughs. I have published some of these approaches in books about cancer (*Bridges of the Bodymind* and *Imagery of Cancer*), autism (*The Autism Answer*), addiction (*PsychoNeuroPlasticity Protocols in Addiction*), intelligence (*The IQ Answer*), post-traumatic stress disorder (*The PTSD Breakthrough*), and stress (*The Stress Answer* and *Retraining the Brain*). I would like to share that data exits for even broader applications that assist our endeavor to build wider avenues of health care.

> **Amyotrophic lateral sclerosis (ALS):** Although we considered there to be no possible cure for this disease, I have noted a patient who used Brent Lewis's recording of *Primitive Truth* to increase his rhythmic energy, Native American peace pipe for exposure to the anti-inflammatory properties of herbs, and imagery that enhanced his immune system's intelligence. These treatments were his choices based on the information he obtained about his disease, and they reversed degeneration to increase his functioning.

Cancer: These participants used a variety of musical CDs, including Brent Lewis's drumming recordings, imagery, strengthening directions, and dancing. Group support was available and family members were supportive in the forms of rituals of recovery.

Stroke: It was noted by other practitioners that stroke victims recovered their walking balance from the use of the BAUD.

Parkinson's: Two cases reported complete relief of their trembling through regaining their arm's motor control with the BAUD.

Our body rhythms and brain rhythms have been measured with precision and are specific to causes and changes. Perhaps more importantly, they can be used "without further harm" and with no side effects, other than feeling enhanced peace and joy. I consider those states to be the true outcomes of wellness.

THE RHYTHM OF CHANGE

We need a revolution of new thought about our health care. There is a parallel concern in climate change, as we run the real risk of killing our world, our home, and ourselves if current behaviors—and the motivations that underlie them—persist any longer. I speculate that the state of our world, whether Earth wellness or human wellness, are in danger because, in modern society, nature and humanity have become disconnected. It is ultimately my vision that we usher in a rebalancing of the human body and of the world's ecosystems simultaneously, as one, because each person's efforts to reset their rhythms into homeostasis and wellness affects the whole.

There are many effective, and even profound, systems of healing in the world. As we bring techniques together that offer consistent clinical and scientific results, and learn to heal ourselves, we can see a revolution in health care that reaches the higher goal of raising the human potential to a deeper sense of spiritual destiny.

Imagine what it would look like if we had wellness centers across the nation in which we could participate in or own health care by strengthening our bodies and minds. We would feel empowered to journey with our challenges on a daily basis, which, over time, increases neurological pathways for full healing, so we can return to our functional lives, rebuild our relationships, and leave illness behind to live in a way that is enhanced by the inner resources we have cultivated. It would be exciting and joyous to feel the rhythms of energy flow through our veins, and we could look in the mirror and see the glisten in our eyes. Even old age would not be seen as a failure of our bodies, rather as another fresh opportunity for self-discovery. Causes and personal missions would blossom, and dreams could be realized.

As you feel the effects of healing rhythms in your life, dare to dream with me and soon we will all realize that, at the core of our being, we have a living drum. It keeps us alive, connects us to others and the universe, including a higher power, and helps us have faith in our dreams. All these things are essential self-empowerments when change—in yourself and in the world—feels difficult. For humankind, nothing offers as much healing as the universal rhythm of our heart.

ACKNOWLEDGMENTS

There are many parents of the concepts in this book, but special acknowledgments go out to those involved in the direct manifestation of the script. First and always, I give thanks to my good and trusted friend, Dr. Phil McGraw, who has been my support and mentor for more than forty-five years. Anthony Haskins has been my muse and collaborator for many projects, and has been invaluable to the depth of research and formulating the final form for massive amounts of data. The person who was instrumental to publication was my favorite writing consultant, Jennifer L. Holder. Friends like Dr. Farrah Khaleghi of Creative Care, and Dr. John Chirban of Harvard, offered their wonderful insights and comments along the way. I especially want to thank Greg White of Great Sounds for his mastery of the musical structure that led to the sounds underlying my research in brain response. I also want to acknowledge Dr. Barbara Peavey, my partner at PNP, and the staff, for their help in pursing the "truth" of how healing rhythms work with patients.

REFERENCES

Alabdulgader, A. A. "Coherence: A Novel Nonpharmacological Modality for Lowering Blood Pressure in Hyerptensive Patients." *Global Advances in Health and Medicine* (2012): 56-64.

"Understand the Facts: Physical Activity Reduces Stress." *Anxiety and Depression Association of America.* https://adaa.org/understanding-anxiety/related-illnesses/other-related-conditions/stress/physical-activity-reduces-st.

Sharma, Amit and Awadhesh Kumar Maurya. "Aggregate Frequencies of Body Organs." *International Journal of Electrical, Electronics and Data Communication* 5 (2017).

Chaouloff, F. (1989). "Physical exercise and brain monoamines: a review." *Acta Physiologica Scandinavica* (1989): 1-13.

Cotman, C. B. "Exercise builds brain health: key roles of growth factor cascades and inflammation." *National*

Center for Biotechnology Information: Trends in Neurosciences (2007): 462-72.

Medical Research Council. "How Eating Feeds into the Body Clock." *Science Daily.* www.sciencedaily.com/releases/2019/04/190425143607.htm.

Crosby, Guy and Adrianna D.T. Fabbri. "A Review of the Impact of Preparation and Cooking on the Nutritional Quality of Vegetables and Legumes." *International Journal of Gastronomy and Food Science* 3 (2016).

Benton, David. "Portion Size: What We Know and What We Need to Know." *Critical Reviews in Food Science and Nutrition* (2015): 988-1004.

Farooq, Muhammad and Edward Sazonov. "Automatic Measurement of Chew Count and Chewing Rate During Food Intake." *Electronics (Basel)* (2016).

Lawlis, G. Frank. *Transpersonal Medicine.* Boston: Shambhala Publications, Inc., 1996.

Lawlis, G. Frank. *PsychoNeuroPlasticity Protocols for Addiction.* Lanham: Rowman & Littlefield, 2015.

Hills, A. P. et al. "'Small changes' to diet and physical activity behaviors for weight management." *Obesity Facts* (2013): 228-238.

Achterberg, Jeanne. *Bridges of the Bodymind: Behavioral Approaches to Health Care.* Champaign: Institute for Personality and Ability Testing, 1980.

Sowndhararaja, Kandhasamy and Songmun Kim. "Influence of Frangrances on Human Psychophysiological Activity: With Special Reference to Human Electroencephalographic Response." *Scientia Pharmaceutica* 84 (2016): 724-75.

King, Kelly. "A Review of the Effects of Guided Imagery on Cancer Patients with Pain." *Complementary Health Practice Review* (2010).

Kjellgren, Annette and Jessica Westman. "Beneficial Effects of Treatment with Sensory Isolation in Flotation-Tank as a Preventive Health-Care Intervention." *BMC Complementary and Alternative Medicine* (2014): 417.

Konnikova, Maria. "Goodnight. Sleep Clean." *New York Times*, January 11, 2014. https://www.nytimes.com/2014/01/12/opinion/sunday/goodnight-sleep-clean.html.

U.S. Army Research Laboratory. "Changes in stress after meditation." *Science Daily.* www.sciencedaily.com/releases/2018/06/180621111955.htm.

Dossey, Larry M. *Prayer is Good Medicine.* New York City: Harper Collins, 1996.

Lilly, J. C. *The Deep Self: Consciousness Exploration in the Isolation Tank.* Nevada City: Gateway Books and Tapes, 1977.

Rider, Mark S and Jeanne Achterberg. "Effects of Music-Assisted Imagery on Neutrophils and Lymphocytes." *Applied Psychophysiology and Biofeedback* (1989): 247-257.

Solleveld, Michelle M. et al. "Age-dependent, lasting effects of methylphenidate on the GABAergic system of ADHD patients." *NeuroImage: Clinical* (2017): 812-818.

Miller, James and George Louis Lindenfield. "Auditory Stimulation Therapy for PTSD." Conference: 88th Annual Scientific Meeting of the Aerospace Medical Association. Denver: ResearchGate, 2017.

Myers, C. A. et al. "Food Cravings and Body Weight: A Conditioning Response." *Current Opinion in Endocrinology, Diabetes, and Obesity* (2018): 298-302.

Nguyen, Jessica and Eric Brymer. "Nature-Based Guided Imagery as an Intervention for State Anxiety." *Frontiers in Psychology* (2018): 9.

Peavey, B. S. et al. "Biofeedback Assisted Relaxation Effects on Phagocytic Capacity." *Biofeedback and Self Regulation* (1985).

"Relaxation Techniques: Breath Control Helps Quell Arrant Stress Response." *Harvard Medical School, Trusted Advice for a Healthier Life.* https://www.health.harvard. edu/mind-and-mood/relaxation-techniques-breath-control-helps-quell-errant-stress-response.

Becker, Robert O. and Gary Selden. *The Body Electric: Electromagnetism and the Foundation of Life.* New York City: William Morrow and Company, Inc., 1985.

Sanders, Laura. "Opioids kill. Here's how an overdose shuts down your body." *Science News,* March 31, 2018. https://www.sciencenews.org/article/ opioid-crisis-overdose-death.

Sedikides, Constantine." Assessment, Enhancement and Verification Determinants of the Self-Evaluation Process." *Journal of Personality and Social Psychology* (1993): 317-338.

Storr, Anthony. *Solitude: A Return to the Self.* New York City: Ballantine Books, 1988.

Storr, Anthony. *Solitude: A Return to the Self.* New York: Ballantine Books, 1988.

Thoma, Myriam V. et al. "The Effect of Music on the Human Stress Response." *PLOS One* (2013).

"Scientists Research Effects of Infrasonic Vibrations in Humans." *National Research Nuclear University* (2016).

Wang, Y. T. et al. "Tai Chi, Yoga, and Qigong as Mind-
	Body Exercises." *Evidence Based Complementary
	and Alternative Medicine* (2017): https://doi.
	org/10.1155/2017/8763915.

Fang, Zhuo et al. "Brain Activation Time-Locked to Sleep
	Spindles Associated With Human Cognitive Abilities."
	Frontiers in Neuroscience (2019).